Get Through

Medical School: 1100 SBAs/BOFs and EMQs

Second edition

Get Through

Medical School: 1100 SBAs/BOFs and EMQs

Second edition

Seema Khan MBBS MRCS MRCGP DRCOG
General Practitioner, Kent

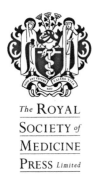

The ROYAL
SOCIETY *of*
MEDICINE
PRESS *Limited*

Published in Great Britain in 2011 by
Hodder Arnold, an imprint of Hodder Education, an Hachette UK company,
338 Euston Road, London NW1 3BH

http://www.hodderarnold.com

First published by The Royal Society of Medicine Press Ltd, 1 Wimpole Street,
London W1G 0AE, UK
The logo of The Royal Society of Medicine is a registered trade mark, which it has licensed to
Hodder Arnold.

Hachette UK's policy is to use papers that are natural, renewable and recyclable products and
made from wood grown in sustainable forests. The logging and manufacturing processes are
expected to conform to the environmental regulations of the country of origin.

Whilst the advice and information in this book are believed to be true and accurate at the date of
going to press, neither the author[s] nor the publisher can accept any legal responsibility or
liability for any errors or omissions that may be made. In particular, (but without limiting the
generality of the preceding disclaimer) every effort has been made to check drug dosages;
however it is still possible that errors have been missed. Furthermore, dosage schedules are
constantly being revised and new side-effects recognized. For these reasons the reader is strongly
urged to consult the drug companies' printed instructions before administering any of the drugs
recommended in this book.

British Library Cataloguing in Publication Data
A catalogue record for this book is available from the British Library

Library of Congress Cataloging-in-Publication Data
A catalog record for this book is available from the Library of Congress

ISBN-13   9781853158667

1 2 3 4 5 6 7 8 9 10

Typeset by TechSet Composition Limited, Salisbury
Printed and bound in the UK by Bell & Bain

What do you think about this book? Or any other Hodder Arnold title?
Please visit our website: www.hodderarnold.com

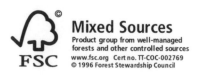

Mixed Sources
Product group from well-managed
forests and other controlled sources
www.fsc.org Cert no. TT-COC-002769
© 1996 Forest Stewardship Council

Contents

Preface

The first edition of *Get Through Medical School*, published in 2003, was one of the first books of its kind on the market. Hugely popular, it was designed to provide medical students with a revision guide based on the changing format of UK medical exams. Since its publication it has successfully helped thousands of students pass their exams and navigate through the challenges presented during junior doctor training.

Several years on, the various UK medical schools have all now adopted their own specific exam formats based on single best answers (SBAs), best of fives (BOFs) and extended matching questions (EMQs). Significant changes have also occurred in the structure of medical training with a 2-year postgraduate foundation programme being introduced in place of the house officer and first year senior house officer years.

The second edition of this book addresses the changes in training and the profession made since the book was first published. The book has been restructured with a number of questions reworded, significantly more detail added in the answer sections and over 100 new questions added. *Get Through Medical School*, second edition, now presents well over 1000 clinically relevant SBAs, BOFs and EMQs across the core curriculum of medicine, surgery, obstetrics and gynaecology, paediatrics and psychiatry. This is a valuable book not only for passing medical school examinations but also for preparing for the clinical scenarios likely to be encountered while practising medicine.

This book is an absolute must for all students serious about successfully getting through medical school and beyond.

SK

Acknowledgement

The author would like to thank Dr Phil Timms, Senior Lecturer in Community Psychiatry, United Medical and Dental Schools, St Thomas' Hospital for his editorial input for the questions on psychiatry.

How to use this book

This section is here to provide some suggestions as to how you can make the most of this book in preparing for your exams. Given that you are in a medical school and have progressed to this stage of higher education means that you are very familiar with and probably fairly good at exams. It is important to remind yourself of this simple fact.

We all know that exam revision requires plenty of time and that it should not be left to the last minute; however, we also know that in reality this is not always going to be possible. This book caters for all students from those who have started their revision early and left themselves plenty of time to work up to an exam to those who have got a couple of weeks to go and are now left with no choice but to get in some last minute focused cramming.

Regardless of which of the two categories you are in, the very first thing you should do is ensure that you know the answers to the following questions:

- What topics will the exam cover?
- When is the exam and how long is it?
- How many questions?
- What is the format and structure of the exam and what style of questions will be used?
- What is the exam marking scheme and what is the pass mark?

These questions will help to shape your revision strategy.

Long-term preparation

If you are going for the long-term exam preparation option then the amount of time that you spend is a very personal thing. Between 6 and 8 weeks is a common timeframe that many people use but this is dependent on (1) the subject matter, (2) the amount of prior knowledge, (3) other commitments over the coming weeks and (4) the number of exams that you have to sit.

Time management is critical. Create a reasonable revision schedule that you know you can achieve and stick to it. Make sure that you get plenty of sleep, eat well and exercise properly; no matter what you think, the absence of any of these three ingredients will significantly reduce your chances of successfully passing/doing well in your exams.

You can use this book to test your knowledge of each of the specialties as you revise them. The questions will test your comprehension and retention of particular topics and the answer sections can be equally important in cementing that understanding and challenging why the other options are incorrect.

Short-term focused cramming

This is not the recommended option but if you have no choice you can certainly use this book to help target last minute revision. Work through the questions and take your time looking at the answers, understanding the justifications given in each case. When the rationale given in the answer sections is unfamiliar, use the questions and options as a basis to target further reading.

Recommended reading

Medicine

British Medical Association, Royal Pharmaceutical Society of Great Britain. *British National Formulary 58*. London: Pharmaceutical Press, 2009.

Fauci AS, Braunwald E, Kasper DL et al. *Harrison's Principles of Internal Medicine*, 17th edn. New York: McGraw-Hill Medical, 2008.

Kumar P, Clark ML. *Kumar and Clark's Clinical Medicine*, 5th edn. London: Saunders, 2009.

Longmore M, Wilkinson I, Turmezei T, Cheung CK. *Oxford Handbook of Clinical Medicine*, 7th edn. Oxford: OUP, 2007.

Resuscitation Council. *Advanced Life Support Course Provider Manual*, 4th edn. London: Resuscitation Council, 2004.

Rubenstein D, Wayne D, Bradley JR. *Lecture Notes on Clinical Medicine*, 6th edn. Oxford: Blackwell Publishing, 2002.

Surgery

Ellis H, Calne R, Watson C. *Lecture Notes on General Surgery*, 11th edn. Oxford: Wiley-Blackwell, 2006.

Harken AH. *Abernathy's Surgical Secrets*, 6th edn. Philadelphia: Mosby, 2008.

Lattimer CR, Lagattolla NRF, Wilson NM. *Key Topics in General Surgery*, 2nd edn. London: Informa Healthcare, 2002.

McLatchie G, Borley N, Chikwe J, eds. *Oxford Handbook of Clinical Surgery*, 3rd edn. Oxford: OUP, 2007.

Roland NJ, McRae RDR, McCombe, eds. *Key Topics in Otolaryngology*, 2nd edn. London: Informa Healthcare, 2000.

Solomon L, Warwick D, Nayagam S. *Apley's System of Orthopaedics and Fractures*, 9th edn. London: Hodder Arnold, 2009.

Unwin, A, Jones K. *Emergency Orthopaedics and Trauma*. Oxford: Butterworth-Heinemann, 1995.

Psychiatry

American Psychiatric Association. *Diagnostic and Statistical Manual of Mental Disorders*, 4th edn. Washington DC: American Psychiatric Association, 2000.

Davies T, Craig T, eds. *ABC of Mental Health*, 2nd edn. Oxford: Wiley-Blackwell, 2009.

Tomb DA. *Psychiatry*, 7th edn. Baltimore: Lippincott, Williams & Wilkins, 2007.

Obstetrics and gynaecology

Chamberlain G, Hamilton-Fairley D. *Lecture Notes on Obstetrics and Gynaecology*. Oxford: Wiley-Blackwell, 1999.

Collier J, Longmore M, Turmezei T, Mafi A. *Oxford Handbook of Clinical Specialties*, 8th edn. Oxford: Oxford University Press, 2009.

Glasier A, Gebbie A. *Handbook of Family Planning and Reproductive Healthcare*, 5th edn. London: Churchill Livingstone, 2007.

Hacker NF, Gambone JC, Hobel CJ. *Hacker and Moore's Essentials of Obstetrics and Gynaecology*, 5th edn. Philadelphia: WB Saunders, 2009.

Paediatrics

Kliegman RM, Behrman RE, Jenson HB, Stanton B. *Nelson Textbook of Pediatrics*. Philadelphia: WB Saunders, 2007.

Lissauer T, Clayden G. *Illustrated Textbook of Paediatrics*, 3rd edn. London: Mosby, 2007.

Abbreviations

AAA	aortic abdominal aneurysm
A&E	accident and emergency department
ABC	airway, breathing and circulation
ABPI	ankle brachial pressure index
ACE	angiotensin-converting enzyme
ACTH	adrenocorticotrophic hormone
ADH	antidiuretic hormone
AIDS	acquired immune deficiency syndrome
ALP	alkaline phosphatase
AMAs	anti-mitochondrial antibodies
ANAs	anti-nuclear antibodies
APTT	activated partial thromboplastin time
ARDS	acute respiratory distress syndrome
ASIS	anterior superior iliac spine
AST	aspartate transaminase
AV	atrioventricular
BCC	basal cell carcinoma
BMI	body mass index
BP	blood pressure
CBD	common bile duct
CBT	cognitive–behavioural therapy
CEA	carcinoembyonic antigen
CIN	cervical invasive neoplasia
CMV	cytomegalovirus
CNS	central nervous system
COC	combination oral contraceptive
COX	cyclo-oxygenase
CPR	cardiopulmonary resuscitation
CREST	Calcinosis, Raynaud's syndrome, Esophageal dysmotility, Sclerodactyly, Telangiectasia
CRP	C-reactive protein
C-section	caesarean section
CSF	cerebrospinal fluid
CT	computed tomography
CTPA	computed tomography pulmonary angiogram
CVA	cerebrovascular accident
CVP	central venous pressure
DIC	disseminated intravascular coagulopathy
DRE	digital rectal examination
dsDNA	double-stranded deoxyribonucleic acid
DVT	deep venous thrombosis
EAA	extrinsic allergic alveolitis
EBV	Epstein–Barr virus
ECG	electrocardiogram
ECT	electroconvulsive treatment
ECV	external cephalic version
EEG	electroencephalogram
ELISA	enzyme-linked immunosorbent assay

EMDR	eye movement desensitization and reprocessing
ENA	extractable nuclear antigen
ENT	ear, nose and throat
ER	oestrogen receptor
ERCP	endoscopic retrograde cholangiopancreatography
ESR	erythrocyte sedimentation rate
EUA	explore under anaesthetic
FBC	full blood count
FNAC	fine-needle aspiration cytology
FSH	follicle-stimulating hormone
G6PD	glucose-6-phosphate dehydrogenase
GCS	Glasgow Coma Scale
GI	gastrointestinal
GnRH	gonadotrophin releasing hormone
GTN	glyceryl trinitrate
HAV	hepatitis A virus
Hb	haemoglobin
HbA1c	glycated haemoglobin
βhCG	β human chorionic gonadotrophin
Hib	*Haemophilus influenzae* type b
HIDA	hepatobiliary iminodiacetic acid
HIV	human immunodeficiency virus
HLA	human leucocyte antigen
HRT	hormone replacement therapy
IADSA	intra-arterial digital subtraction angiography
I&D	investigate and identify
INR	international normalized ratio
ITP	idiopathic thrombocytopenic purpura
IU	international units
IUCD	intrauterine contraceptive device
IUGR	intrauterine growth retardation
IUS	intrauterine system
JVP	jugular venous pressure
KUB	kidney, ureter and bladder
LDH	lactate dehydrogenase
LDL	low-density lipoprotein
LFT	liver function test
LH	luteinizing hormone
MAOI	monoamine oxidase inhibitor
MCAD	medium-chain acyl-CoA dehydrogenase
MCHC	mean corpuscular haemoglobin concentration
MC&S	microscopy, culture and sensitivity
MCH	mean corpuscular haemoglobin
MCV	mean corpuscular volume
MDMA	3,4-methylenedioxymethamphetamine
MEN	multiple endocrine neoplasia
MI	myocardial infarction
MMSE	Mini-Mental State Examination
MRCP	magnetic resonance cholangiopancreatography
MRI	magnetic resonance imaging
MSA	multi-system atrophy

MSU	midstream specimen of urine
NSAID	non-steroidal anti-inflammatory drug
OCD	obsessive–compulsive disorder
OGD	oesophagogastroduodenoscopy
OGTT	oral glucose tolerance test
$PaCO_2$	partial arterial CO_2 pressure
PaO_2	partial arterial O_2 pressure
PBC	primary biliary cirrhosis
PCA	patient-controlled analgesia
PCO	polycystic ovary
PCOS	polycystic ovarian syndrome
PE	pulmonary embolism
PEA	pulseless electrical activity
PEFR	peak expiratory flow rate
PEG	percutaneous endoscopic gastrostomy
PET	positron emission tomography
PID	pelvic inflammatory disease
POP	progesterone-only pill
PSA	prostate-specific antigen
PTH	parathyroid hormone
PTSD	post-traumatic stress disorder
PTT	prothrombin time
RAD	right axis deviation
RIF	right iliac fossa
RSV	respiratory syncytial virus
RTA	road traffic accident
RVH	right ventricular hypertrophy
SCC	squamous cell carcinoma
SIADH	syndrome of inappropriate antidiuretic hormone secretion
SLE	systemic lupus erythematosus
SSRI	selective serotonin reuptake inhibitor
STI	sexually transmitted infection
SVC	superior vena cava
SVD	spontaneous vaginal delivery
SVT	supraventricular tachycardia
T_4	thyroxine
TB	tuberculosis
TCA	tricyclic antidepressant
TdT	terminal deoxyribonucleotidyltransferase
TFT	thyroid function test
TIA	transient ischaemic accident
TIBC	total iron-binding capacity
TOP	termination of pregnancy
tPA	tissue plasminogen activator
TRH	thyroid-releasing hormone
TSH	thyroid-stimulating hormone
TTP	thrombotic thrombocytopenic purpura
TURP	transurethral resection of the prostate
U&Es	urea and electrolytes
UPT	urine pregnancy test

URTI	upper respiratory tract infection
UTI	urinary tract infection
VDRL	Venereal Diseases Research Laboratory
$\dot{V}/\dot{Q}$	ventilation–perfusion
vWF	von Willebrand's factor
WBC	white blood cell count

To Faheem and all the family, with love

1. MEDICINE

1. Medicine: SBA/BOF Questions

In these questions candidates must select one answer only.

1) A 50-year-old man complains of hardness of hearing and dyspnoea. He is noted to have a nasal septal perforation and a blood pressure of 140/90 mmHg. His urinalysis shows red cells, protein and casts. The chest radiograph reveals opacities. The most likely diagnosis is:

   a. Tuberculosis
   b. Amyloidosis
   c. Goodpasture's syndrome
   d. Acute tubulointerstitial nephritis
   e. Wegener's granulomatosis

2) Pulseless electrical activity (PEA) in a cardiac arrest may be associated with all of the following EXCEPT:

   a. Cardiac tamponade
   b. Thromboembolism
   c. Malignant hyperpyrexia
   d. Hypokalaemia
   e. Ruptured aortic aneurysm

3) A 75-year-old man with type 1 diabetes mellitus presents with a unilateral facial nerve palsy and severe earache. On auroscopic examination, he has granulation tissue deep in the external auditory meatus. The most likely diagnosis is:

   a. Bell's palsy
   b. Sarcoidosis
   c. Facial nerve schwannoma
   d. Otitis externa complicated by local osteomyelitis (malignant otitis externa)
   e. Suppurative otitis media

4) A 70-year-old woman presents with recent onset of urinary incontinence. The most appropriate initial investigation is:

   a. Mid-stream urine (MSU) sample for dipstick
   b. Urodynamics
   c. FBC
   d. Serum urea and electrolytes
   e. MSU for culture and sensitivities

5) A 50-year-old woman with type 2 diabetes mellitus presents with fever and a well-defined dusky-red erythematous eruption over the left side of her face. The most likely organism would be:

   a. *Staphylococcus aureus*
   b. Group B streptococcus
   c. Group A streptococcus
   d. Herpes zoster virus
   e. Herpes simplex virus

6) The following diseases are associated with the Epstein–Barr virus EXCEPT:

   a. Craniopharyngioma
   b. Burkitt's lymphoma
   c. Sinonasal tumours
   d. Glandular fever
   e. Hodgkin's lymphoma

7) A 44-year-old woman complains of headaches and nosebleeds. Blood pressure is 160/100 mmHg in the right arm and 130/80 mmHg in the left arm. She complains of cold legs and has delayed radiofemoral pulses. The most likely diagnosis would be:

   a. Acromegaly
   b. Marfan's syndrome
   c. Coarctation of the aorta
   d. Kawasaki's disease
   e. Takayasu's arteritis

8) A 55-year-old farmer complains of dry cough, exertional dyspnoea, joint pains and weight loss. He is noted to have finger clubbing. On a chest radiograph there is bilateral diffuse reticulonodular shadowing at the bases. The most likely diagnosis is:

   a. Bronchial carcinoma
   b. Bronchiectasis
   c. Cryptogenic fibrosing alveolitis
   d. Mesothelioma
   e. Extrinsic allergic alveolitis

9) A 45-year-old woman presents with pruritus and jaundice. She complains of dry eyes and mouth. The most discriminating investigation would be:

   a. Anti-mitochondrial antibodies
   b. Antinuclear antibody
   c. Serum bilirubin and liver function tests
   d. Hepatitis B surface antigen
   e. Smooth muscle antibody

10) An 80-year-old woman complains of sudden painless loss of vision in her right eye. She has facial pain on chewing. The most likely diagnosis is:

   a. Acute glaucoma
   b. Retinal detachment
   c. Cranial arteritis
   d. Basilar migraine
   e. Optic neuritis

11) A 13-year-old girl presents with a painful and swollen knee. There is no history of trauma. A tender lump is palpated over the tibial tuberosity. The most likely diagnosis would be:

   a. Osteomyelitis
   b. Chondromalacia patella
   c. Juvenile rheumatoid arthritis
   d. Osteosarcoma
   e. Osgood–Schlatter disease

12) The following pairs of neurovascular structures and injuries are correctly paired EXCEPT:

   a. Tibial nerve – proximal fibula fracture
   b. Sciatic nerve – posterior dislocation of the hip
   c. Median nerve – Smith's wrist fracture
   d. Axillary nerve – fracture to humeral neck
   e. Brachial artery – supracondylar fracture of the humerus

13) An 18 year old known to have asthma presents with severe wheezing, a respiratory rate of 30 and a pulse of 120. She is using her accessory muscles and appears distressed. She is apyrexial. The most appropriate initial management would be:

   a. Intramuscular adrenaline
   b. Oxygen and nebulized salbutamol
   c. Intravenous hydrocortisone
   d. Endotracheal intubation
   e. Intravenous penicillin

14) A 25-year-old woman is brought to the accident and emergency department (A&E) by ambulance having sustained gross maxillofacial deformities after a high-speed road traffic accident. She is now agitated and hypoxic despite high-concentration oxygen having been administered by facemask by the paramedics. The most appropriate immediate intervention is:

   a. Endotracheal intubation
   b. Nasopharyngeal airway
   c. Oropharyngeal airway
   d. Cricothyroidotomy
   e. Laryngeal mask airway

15) The following pulse patterns are correctly matched with their disorders EXCEPT:

   a. Pulsus alternans – left ventricular failure
   b. Pulsus paradoxus – cardiac tamponade
   c. Pulsus bisferiens – hypertrophic obstructive cardiomyopathy
   d. Pulsus parvus et tardus (small volume, slow rising) – aortic regurgitation
   e. Dicrotic pulse – dilated cardiomyopathy

16) A 16-year old girl presents with an anterior neck mass. It moves on protrusion of her tongue. Thyroid radionuclide scan shows no uptake in the midline. The most likely diagnosis is:

   a. Lingual thyroid
   b. Hashimoto's thyroiditis
   c. Thyroglossal cyst
   d. Thyroid follicular adenoma
   e. Reidel's thyroiditis

17) A 40-year-old man presents with progressive confusion and tremor. On examination, he has extensor plantar reflexes. The most useful investigation would be:

   a. HIV serology
   b. CT scan
   c. Drug levels
   d. Mantoux test
   e. VDRL

18) A 45-year-old man with a history of epilepsy presents with several weeks of fluctuating levels of consciousness. On examination his pupils are unequal. The most discriminating investigation is:

   a. HIV serology
   b. CT scan
   c. EEG
   d. Drug levels
   e. Lumbar puncture

19) A 20-year-old heroin addict presents with weight loss, diarrhoea and confusion. On examination he has purple papules on his legs. The most useful investigation is:

   a. Echocardiogram
   b. Blood cultures
   c. HIV serology
   d. Chest radiograph
   e. Drug levels

20) Coeliac disease is associated with all of the following EXCEPT:

   a. Vitamin B_{12} deficiency
   b. HLA DR3
   c. Dermatitis herpetiformis
   d. Steatorrhoea
   e. Lymphoma

21) A 60-year-old man presents with acute onset of confusion and restlessness; he walks with a broad-based gait. On examination there is nystagmus and lateral rectus palsies bilaterally. There is alcoholic fetor. The most likely diagnosis would be:

   a. Alcohol withdrawal
   b. Folic acid deficiency
   c. Subarachnoid haemorrhage
   d. Subdural haematoma
   e. Wernicke–Korsakoff syndrome

22) A 40-year-old woman complains of disabling joint pains. On examination you note scaly plaques over her anterior shins and knees. She has tried diclofenac for the arthralgia and wonders if there is any connection with the rash. The most useful treatment for her joints now would be:

   a. Oral prednisolone
   b. Methotrexate
   c. Co-dydramol
   d. Topical 0.5% hydrocortisone
   e. Dithranol 0.1% cream

23) A 50-year-old man presents to A&E complaining of 30 minutes of severe crushing midchest pain with no relief from GTN. He has a history of angina. Pulse is 105 and BP 115/60. A 12-lead ECG shows normal sinus rhythm. The first drug to administer would be:

   a. Morphine
   b. Oxygen
   c. Gaviscon
   d. Streptokinase
   e. Atropine

24) A 40-year-old woman with a history of angina presents with severe chest pain for 30 minutes. Pulse is 45 and blood pressure 80/60. A 12-lead ECG shows third-degree heart block. The first drug to administer would be:

   a. Lidocaine
   b. Atropine
   c. Adrenaline
   d. Procainamide
   e. Amiodarone

25) A 40-year-old patient is brought to A&E by ambulance in pulseless electrical activity (PEA). You are told that he was given adrenaline. The next step would be to:

a. Evaluate for reversible causes
b. Defibrillate with 200 J
c. Administer verapamil
d. Administer amiodarone
e. Administer morphine

26) A 70-year-old woman presents with progressive dysphagia and food regurgitation. On examination she has halitosis and a small lump on the left side of her neck. The most likely diagnosis is:

a. Achalasia
b. Branchial cyst
c. Diffuse oesophageal spasm
d. Pharyngeal pouch
e. Myasthenia gravis

27) A 40-year-old woman on carbamazepine for trigeminal neuralgia now complains of severe dizziness. The drug that may have potentiated the side effects of carbamazepine is:

a. the combined oral contraceptive pill
b. erythromycin
c. chloramphenicol
d. omeprazole
e. thiazide diuretics

28) The most common type of thyroid carcinoma is:

a. Follicular
b. Anaplastic
c. Medullary
d. Squamous
e. Papillary

29) A 40-year-old woman presents with fatigue, dyspnoea and paraesthesiae. On examination she has a red tongue. Blood film shows hypersegmented neutrophils, an Hb of 9 and a mean corpuscular volume (MCV) of 120 fL. The most likely diagnosis is:

a. Vitamin B_{12} deficiency
b. Iron deficiency
c. Coeliac disease
d. Sideroblastic anaemia
e. Hypothyroidism

30) An 18-year-old young women, who recently started the combined oral contraceptive pill on holiday in Kenya, complains of colicky abdominal pain, vomiting and fever. Urine is positive for red blood cells and protein. She develops progressive weakness in her extremities. The most likely diagnosis is:

a. Acute pyelonephritis
b. Acute intermittent porphyria
c. Ureteric calculus
d. Malaria
e. Systemic lupus erythematosus

31) A 75-year-old man presents with dyspnoea and chest pain. His pulse rate is 120 and he is extremely agitated. His arterial blood gas reveals low arterial oxygen and low CO_2. His ECG shows S wave in I, Q and T waves in III, and T-wave inversion in leads V1–3. The most likely diagnosis is:

a. Myocardial infarction
b. Pulmonary embolism
c. Acute pericarditis
d. Cardiac tamponade
e. Pneumothorax

32) A 40-year-old actor with type 1 diabetes mellitus is started on propranolol for stage fright. He collapses on stage. He has not changed his insulin regimen. Serum glucose is 1.5 mmol/L. The most beneficial advice that you would offer him after treatment would be:

a. Discontinue propranolol
b. Carry a chocolate bar
c. Decrease his Humulin insulin
d. Decrease his Actrapid insulin
e. Carry glucagon

33) A 40-year-old woman complains of intolerance to cold weather and cold running water. On examination you note that she has a beaked nose, radial furrowing of the lips and facial telangiectasias. On examination of her hands you notice sausage-like digits and tapered fingers. The most discriminating investigation to establish her diagnosis is:

a. Anticentromere antinuclear antibody
b. Rheumatoid factor
c. FBC
d. Chest radiograph
e. Barium swallow

34) Sites of a carcinoid tumour include all of the following EXCEPT the:

   a. Appendix
   b. Terminal ileum
   c. Bronchus
   d. Oesophagus
   e. Rectum

35) Stevens–Johnson syndrome is associated with all of the following drugs EXCEPT:

   a. Penicillin
   b. Sulphonamides
   c. Oral contraceptives
   d. Thiazide diuretics
   e. Salicylates

36) A 32-year-old boxer presents with headache, drowsiness, seizures and a rising blood pressure. The next most appropriate investigation is:

   a. Blood alcohol level
   b. Lumbar puncture
   c. CT scan of the head
   d. Blood glucose
   e. Blood cultures

37) A 55-year-old woman complains of sudden, severe, central abdominal pain radiating to her back and vomiting. She prefers to sit forward on her stretcher. Temperature is 39°C, BP 100/60 and pulse 112. On examination she has a markedly tender epigastrium and a bruise over the left flank. She has a history of gallstones. She denies smoking or drinking alcohol. She takes HRT. The best initial investigation would be:

   a. Plain abdominal radiograph
   b. Serum bilirubin and liver function tests
   c. Serum amylase
   d. FBC
   e. Abdominal ultrasonography

38) A 20-year-old man presents with a 4-day history of itching in both eyes. On examination there is bilateral lid oedema and a watery clear discharge. The most likely diagnosis is:

   a. Episcleritis
   b. Corneal abrasion
   c. Trichiasis
   d. Blepharitis
   e. Allergic conjunctivitis

39) A 75-year-old Asian woman presents with a 5-month history of tiredness and breathlessness particularly on exertion. On examination there is bilateral pitting oedema and fine crepitations bibasally. The most likely diagnosis is:

a. Malignancy
b. Chronic fatigue syndrome
c. Liver failure
d. Congestive cardiac failure
e. Tuberculosis

40) A 55-year-old man is found to have a fasting venous plasma glucose level of 6.3 mmol/L. What is the next step in management:

a. Commence glitazone
b. Fasting glucose test
c. Glucose tolerance test
d. Dietary advice
e. Urine dipstick

41) A 17-year-old boy presents with pain on swallowing. On examination he has trismus, palatal petechiae and enlarged tonsils. His sclerae are jaundiced. The most likely causative organism is:

a. *Streptococcus pneumoniae*
b. Hepatitis B virus
c. Epstein–Barr virus
d. Herpes simplex virus
e. *Clostridium tetani*

42) A 20-year-old woman presents with recurrent epistaxis. She admits to having heavy periods. Her BP is 90/60 and pulse 100. There are bruises of different ages over her extremities but no splenomegaly. Test results are as follows:

White cell count	83×10^9/L
Hb	11.5 g/dL
Platelets	149×10^9/L
Bleeding time	Prolonged
Antinuclear antibody	Negative

The most likely diagnosis is:

a. Non-accidental injury
b. Systemic lupus erythematosus
c. Idiopathic thrombocytopenic purpura (ITP)
d. Thrombotic thrombocytopenic purpura (TTP)
e. Sickle cell disease

43) A 45-year-old woman presents with severe itching, pale stools and dark urine. On examination there is darkened skin pigmentation, xanthelasma and hepatomegaly. Test results are as follows:

Serum bilirubin	15 mmol/L
Serum alkaline phosphatase	400 (30–300) IU/L
AST	40 (5–35) IU/L

Diagnosis would best be confirmed by:

a. Serum antimitochondrial antibody
b. Hepatitis virology
c. Liver biopsy
d. Kveim's test
e. Abdominal ultrasonography

44) A 60-year-old man presents with increasing abdominal girth. On examination you elicit shifting dullness. The ascitic fluid tap reveals straw-coloured fluid containing 50 g/L of protein and elevated LDH. It contains 1000 WBCs/mm^3 (no lymphocytes) and many red cells are present. Serum total protein is 40 g/L. The most likely diagnosis is:

a. Cirrhosis
b. Tuberculosis
c. Malignancy
d. Pancreatitis
e. Hepatic vein obstruction

45) A 20-year-old homosexual man presents with proctalgia and bloody anal discharge. The most likely organism is:

a. Human papillomavirus
b. Chlamydia trachomatis
c. Neisseria gonorrhoeae
d. Haemophilus ducreyi
e. Treponema pallidum

46) A 40-year-old long-stay patient in a psychiatric hospital presents with fever, abdominal pain, dry cough and worsening confusion. Blood tests reveal neutrophilia, lymphopenia and hyponatraemia. A chest radiograph shows right-sided lobar consolidation. The most likely diagnosis is:

a. Tuberculosis
b. Streptococcal pneumonia
c. Legionella pneumonia
d. Klebsiella pneumonia
e. Staphylococcal pneumonia

47) A 50-year-old man with schizophrenia presents with drooling saliva and involuntary chewing movements. He walks with a shuffling gait. The most likely diagnosis is:

a. Parkinson's disease
b. Extrapyramidal side effect of medication
c. Autonomic side effect of medication
d. Anticholinergic side effect of medication
e. Lithium toxicity

48) A 40-year-old man presents with numbness and tingling sensation in his feet. He is noted to have distal sensory loss and absent ankle-jerk reflexes. The knee-jerk reflexes are exaggerated. He drinks heavily and smokes cigars. His blood pressure is 160/90 with a pulse of 90. A full blood count reveals a macrocytic megaloblastic anaemia. The most likely diagnosis is:

a. Syringomyelia
b. Tabes dorsalis
c. Wernicke–Korsakoff syndrome
d. Vitamin B_6 deficiency
e. Subacute combined degeneration of the cord

49) A 30-year-old man presents with a brown discoloured toenail. On examination there is nail pitting and brown pigmentation at the base of the great toenail and cuticle. He states that the colour started under the nail and has spread down to his nailbed. The most likely diagnosis is:

a. Subungal haematoma
b. Psoriasis
c. Paronychia
d. Melanoma
e. Onychomycosis

50) A 40-year-old woman presents with a right-sided pleural effusion and ascites. Abdominal ultrasonography reveals a left ovarian mass. The most likely diagnosis is:

a. Pseudomyxoma peritonei
b. Meigs' syndrome
c. Budd–Chiari syndrome
d. Nephrotic syndrome
e. Tuberculosis

51) A 30-year-old man presents with a tender swollen testicle. He states that he was bumped in the groin while playing sports. On examination the borders of the testicle are irregular, and the testicle is heavy and woody. There is no associated lymphadenopathy. He is also noted to have gynaecomastia. There are no external signs of trauma. In this age group, the most likely diagnosis is:

a. Testicular torsion
b. Epididymo-orchitis
c. Seminoma
d. Teratoma
e. Testicular haematoma

52) A 45-year-old male psychiatric patient with long-term bipolar disorder presents with vomiting, muscle twitching and tremor. He was started on bendrofluazide recently and self-prescribes ibuprofen for headaches. His BP is 90/50. His gait is ataxic. He then starts fitting. The drug most likely to be responsible is:

a. Lithium
b. Phenothiazine
c. Benzodiazepine
d. Ecstasy (MDMA)
e. Ibuprofen

53) A 60-year-old man presents acutely with vertigo and vomiting. On neurological examination there is right facial numbness, an ipsilateral ataxia of the arms and legs and a contralateral loss of pain and temperature sense. The most likely diagnosis is:

a. Posterior cerebral artery infarction
b. Middle cerebral artery infarction
c. Anterior cerebral artery infarction
d. Posteroinferior cerebellar artery infarction
e. Vertebrobasilar ischaemia

54) A 60-year-old man presents with persistent fever, profuse watery diarrhoea and crampy abdominal pain for the past week. He has just completed treatment for osteomyelitis. Proctosigmoidoscopy reveals erythematous ulcerations and yellowish-white plaques. The most likely diagnosis is:

a. Ulcerative colitis
b. Crohn's disease
c. Pseudomembranous colitis
d. Viral gastroenteritis
e. *Clostridium perfringens* enterocolitis

55) You are on ward rounds and notice that a young patient is coughing briskly. He has just been started on benzylpenicillin for acute tonsillitis complicated by trismus. He states that he does not know if he is allergic to any drugs. He becomes short of breath. His pulse is 110 beats/min and he now cannot complete sentences. The most appropriate management for this patient would be:

a. Administer adrenaline of a 1:10 000 solution intravenously
b. Administer adrenaline intramuscularly for suspected new-onset asthma
c. Administer oxygen and give nebulized salbutamol
d. Administer oxygen and adrenaline of a 1:1000 solution intramuscularly for suspected anaphylaxis
e. Administer oxygen and give intravenous hydrocortisone for anaphylactic shock

56) A 45-year-old obese man is noted to have glycosuria. He has no symptoms. Diabetes is confirmed on an oral glucose tolerance test. The most appropriate management for this patient is:

a. Commence biguanide
b. Commence sulphonylurea
c. Advise on diet and exercise
d. Commence on Humulin and Actrapid insulin
e. Admit to hospital

57) A 45-year-old man with well-controlled type 1 diabetes is prescribed captopril for hypertension. He has a history of intermittent claudication and has rest pain. There is +++ proteinuria. Urea and creatinine are elevated. On examination there is an abdominal bruit. The most likely diagnosis is:

a. Diabetic nephropathy
b. Focal segmental glomerulosclerosis
c. Renal artery stenosis
d. Membranous glomerulonephritis
e. Renal cholesterol embolism

58) A 20-year-old man presents with buttock pain radiating down both legs and heel pain. On examination he has marked kyphosis and limitation of chest expansion. ESR and CRP were raised. The most likely diagnosis is:

a. Lumbar disc prolapse
b. Sacroiliitis
c. Spondylolisthesis
d. Spinal stenosis
e. Ankylosing spondylitis

59) A 42-year-old woman presents with repeated episodes of fluctuating hearing loss, vertigo and tinnitus lasting hours over the past few months. The cause of her vertigo is:

a. Migraine
b. Hyperventilation
c. Acoustic neuroma
d. Ménière's disease
e. Acute vestibular neuronitis

60) The definitive investigation to diagnose a pulmonary embolism is:

a. Pulmonary arteriography
b. Ventilation–perfusion isotope scintigraphy
c. Computed tomography pulmonary angiogram (CTPA)
d. A 12-lead ECG
e. Posteroanterior and lateral chest radiographs

61) Which one of the following drugs is absolutely contraindicated in patients with asthma?

a. Adenosine
b. Atenolol
c. Adrenaline
d. Verapamil
e. Bendrofluazide

62) A 70-year-old man complains of flashing lights and floaters in his left eye for the past month and now complains of painless loss of vision in his left eye. The most likely diagnosis is:

a. Central retinal artery occlusion
b. Central retinal vein occlusion
c. Optic neuritis
d. Retinal detachment
e. Macular degeneration

63) A 30-year-old man with HIV presents with sudden bilateral painless loss of vision. The most likely cause is:

a. Kaposi's sarcoma
b. Candidiasis
c. *Chlamydia trachomatis*
d. Cytomegalovirus retinitis
e. Gonococcal infection

64) A 50-year-old man presents to A&E with repeated fits. Plasma sodium is 112 mmol/L and urine osmolality is 550 mosmol/kg. He is well hydrated. On his chest radiograph there is a cannon-ball lesion. He smokes 20 cigarettes a day and drinks spirits daily. The most likely diagnosis is:

a. SIADH (syndrome of inappropriate antidiuretic hormone secretion)
b. Addison's disease
c. Liver cirrhosis
d. Renal failure
e. Diabetes insipidus

65) The cause of gradual bilateral loss of vision is least likely to be:

a. Cataract
b. Optic atrophy
c. Diabetic retinopathy
d. Chronic glaucoma
e. Choroiditis

66) A 60-year-old man presents with chest pain and sudden onset of atrial fibrillation with a heart rate of 160/min. The most appropriate management would be:

a. Oxygen, heparin and synchronized DC shock
b. Oxygen, heparin, intravenous amiodarone
c. Oxygen, heparin, warfarin
d. Oxygen, β blockers
e. Oxygen, intravenous digoxin

67) A 65-year-old man presents with an acute myocardial infarction with a new left bundle-branch block. He had a haemorrhagic stroke a year ago. He is given 100% oxygen, diamorphine, metoclopramide, GTN and aspirin. The next most appropriate management is:

a. Intravenous glycoprotein IIb/IIIa inhibitor
b. Thrombolytic therapy with streptokinase
c. Coronary artery bypass surgery
d. Percutaneous transluminal coronary angioplasty
e. Continuous infusion of heparin

68) Which one of the following drugs may induce a psychosis similar to paranoid schizophrenia?

a. Heroin
b. Ecstasy (MDMA)
c. Amphetamine
d. Cocaine
e. Barbiturates

69) Typhoid fever is associated with all of the following EXCEPT:

   a. Bowel perforation
   b. Splenomegaly
   c. Ulceration of Peyer's patches
   d. Non-blanching maculopapular rash
   e. Osteomyelitis

70) A 20-year-old woman presents with a BP of 170/100. On examination she has impalpable peripheral pulses, although systolic murmurs are auscultated above and below her clavicle. She also complains of diminishing vision and syncopal episodes. Her ESR is 50 mm/h. The most likely diagnosis is:

   a. Thrombangiitis obliterans
   b. Coarctation of the aorta
   c. Kawasaki's disease
   d. Takayasu's syndrome
   e. Raynaud's disease

71) A 35-year-old intravenous drug abuser presents with right upper quadrant abdominal pain. On examination he has peripheral oedema, ascites and a pulsatile liver. On chest auscultation he has a pansystolic murmur along the left sternal border. The most likely diagnosis is:

   a. Tricuspid regurgitation
   b. Pulmonary regurgitation
   c. Pulmonary stenosis
   d. Mitral regurgitation
   e. Tricuspid stenosis

72) A 50-year-old woman presents with fever, headache, left eye pain and blurry vision. She states that she has just recovered from a cold. On examination she has a swollen left eyelid, mild proptosis and diminished visual acuity. She is unable to move her eye. The most likely diagnosis is:

   a. Orbital cellulitis
   b. Giant-cell arteritis
   c. Sinusitis
   d. Choroiditis
   e. Cavernous sinus thrombosis

73) A 60-year-old woman presents with progressive forgetfulness and mood changes. She has a shuffling gait. A CT scan of the head shows cortical atrophy and enlarged ventricles. Histology shows senile plaques and neurofibrillary tangles. The most likely diagnosis is:

   a. Wernicke–Korsakoff syndrome
   b. Parkinson's disease
   c. Alzheimer's disease
   d. Variant Creutzfeldt–Jakob disease
   e. Multi-infarct dementia

74) A 20-year-old college student presents with headache and dry cough. The chest radiograph shows left lower lobe consolidation. White cell count is normal. Cold agglutinins are detected. The most likely pathogen is:

    a. *Streptococcus pneumoniae*
    b. *Klebsiella sp.*
    c. *Mycoplasma pneumoniae*
    d. *Haemophilus influenzae*
    e. *Legionella pneumophila*

75) A 25-year-old man presents with weakness and numbness in his lower legs. He has just recovered from a recent chest infection. On examination deep tendon reflexes are absent and sensation is also lost. CSF from a lumbar puncture shows a normal cell count and glucose but raised protein level. The most likely diagnosis is:

    a. Mumps
    b. Sarcoidosis
    c. AIDS
    d. Guillain–Barré syndrome
    e. Refsum's disease

76) A 40-year-old man presents with dysphagia and epigastric pain relieved by food and antacids. On examination he has a palpable epigastric mass, a palpable supraclavicular lymph node and acanthosis nigricans. The most likely diagnosis is:

    a. Oesophageal squamous cell carcinoma
    b. Duodenal ulcer
    c. Peptic stricture of oesophagogastric junction
    d. Gastric adenocarcinoma
    e. Pancreatic carcinoma

77) A 17-year-old girl presents with meningism and conjunctival petechiae. The CSF is turbid with an abundance of polymorphs and protein. Gram-negative cocci are isolated. The most likely organism is:

    a. *Neisseria meningitidis*
    b. *Neisseria gonorrhoeae*
    c. Group B streptococcus
    d. *Haemophilus influenzae*
    e. *Streptococcus pneumoniae*

78) A 22-year-old man presents with fever, sweating, particularly at night, pruritus and weight loss. On examination he has palpable, painless, cervical lymph nodes and no skin manifestations. The most appropriate investigation would be:

    a. FBC
    b. Lymph node biopsy
    c. Chest radiograph
    d. CT scan of the neck and mediastinum
    e. Mantoux test

79) The most likely diagnosis is:

   a. Tuberculosis
   b. Non-Hodgkin's lymphoma
   c. Hodgkin's lymphoma
   d. Acute lymphoblastic leukaemia
   e. Chronic lymphocytic leukaemia

80) A 40-year-old woman complains of intolerance to cold weather and cold running water. On examination you note that she has a beaked nose, radial furrowing of the lips and facial telangiectasias. On examination of her hands you notice sausage-like digits and tapered fingers. The most likely diagnosis is:

   a. SLE
   b. Sjögren's syndrome
   c. Systemic sclerosis
   d. Rheumatoid arthritis
   e. Dermatomyositis

81) A 50-year-old renal transplant recipient on immunosuppressive therapy with ciclosporin, azathioprine and prednisolone is most at risk of developing:

   a. Squamous cell carcinoma of the skin
   b. Basal cell carcinoma of the skin
   c. Lymphoma
   d. Liver failure
   e. Leukaemia

82) A 25-year-old man back from hitchhiking through South America a fortnight ago now presents with explosive, watery, foul-smelling diarrhoea and weight loss. On examination he has abdominal distension. His stools are greasy and contain mucus. The most likely diagnosis is:

   a. Shigella dysentery
   b. Giardiasis
   c. Amoebic dysentery
   d. Crohn's disease
   e. Cystic fibrosis

83) Choice of antibiotic would be:

   a. Ciprofloxacin
   b. Penicillin
   c. Tetracycline
   d. Metronidazole
   e. Erythromycin

84) A 25-year-old man presents to A&E with repeated fits. He smells of alcohol and has jaw trismus. The most appropriate management is:

   a. Give 100 mg intravenous thiamine
   b. Give 50 mL of 50% glucose intravenously
   c. Give 10 mg diazepam i.v. over 2 min
   d. Insert a Guedel oropharyngeal airway and prepare for endotracheal intubation
   e. Insert a nasopharyngeal airway and administer oxygen

85) A 55-year-old man presents with an acutely painful swollen right knee. He was recently prescribed bendrofluazide for mild hypertension. The most useful investigation would be:

   a. FBC and ESR
   b. Viral antibodies including parvovirus
   c. Antinuclear antibody and rheumatoid factor
   d. Aspirate of joint effusion for Gram stain and culture
   e. Aspirate of joint effusion for polarized light microscopy

86) A 17-year-old man with known sickle cell disease presents with severe lower back pain. He has a history of seizures. Initial management should include all of the following EXCEPT:

   a. Give oxygen at 4 L/min via a facemask
   b. Start intravenous fluids
   c. Give pethidine 150 mg i.m. every 2 h until the pain settles
   d. Give morphine 1–2 mg i.v. every 2–3 min until the pain settles
   e. Lumbar spine and pelvic radiograph

87) A 55-year-old intoxicated man is brought to A&E by the police. He is confused and aggressive. There are no external signs of head trauma. His BP is 140/90 and heart rate 110, and he is pale. He has palmar erythema, tremors and smells of alcohol. The initial most useful investigation for this man is:

   a. Blood alcohol level
   b. Head CT scan
   c. γ-Glutamyltransferase
   d. Blood glucose
   e. Clotting screen

88) A 25-year-old man presents to A&E with sudden onset of severe lower back pain that radiates down his right leg. On examination he is noted to have scoliosis of the spine, limited spinal flexion, restricted straight-leg raise, limited hip movements and sensory loss over the dorsum of the right foot. The most likely diagnosis is:

   a. Spondylolisthesis
   b. Ankylosing spondylitis
   c. Acute cord compression
   d. Spondylosis
   e. Lumbar disc prolapse

89) A 35-year-old man presents with progressive weakness in his limbs over the past few days. He had a chest infection 2 weeks before. On examination he has proximal muscle wasting, hypotonia and absent deep tendon reflexes. Lumbar puncture results are:

Cells	4/mL lymphocytes
Chloride	110 mmol/L
Glucose	3.5 mmol/L
Protein	3 g/L

The most likely diagnosis is:

a. Poliomyelitis
b. Botulism
c. Guillain–Barré syndrome
d. AIDS
e. Subacute combined degeneration of the cord

90) The most useful step in guiding management would be:

a. Pulse oximetry
b. Chest radiograph
c. Nerve conduction studies
d. Serial vital capacity
e. Serial peak flow measurement

91) A 60-year-old obese man presents complaining of recurrent abdominal pain radiating to the back and made worse by eating and bending over. Antacids relieve the pain. He smokes 20 cigarettes a day and drinks spirits daily. The most useful investigation would be:

a. Oesophagogastroduodenoscopy (OGD)
b. Double-contrast barium meal
c. *Helicobacter pylori* breath test
d. Abdominal radiograph
e. Abdominal CT scan

92) The following conditions are associated with short stature EXCEPT:

a. Achondroplasia
b. Hypopituitarism
c. Rickets
d. Crohn's disease
e. Klinefelter's syndrome

93) A 30-year-old man presents with crampy abdominal pain, diarrhoea and weight loss. On examination: temperature 39°C, no lymphadenopathy. Barium meal reveals a stricture in the terminal ileum. The most likely diagnosis is:

a. Tuberculosis
b. Crohn's disease
c. Ulcerative colitis
d. Lymphoma
e. Coeliac disease

94) A 30-year-old man presents with a unilateral facial nerve palsy that involves his forehead. Possible causes include the following EXCEPT:

a. Bell's palsy
b. Ramsay–Hunt syndrome
c. Acoustic neuroma
d. Cerebrovascular accident
e. Parotid tumour

95) On general examination the man has coarse oily skin and a prominent supraorbital ridge. He has widely spaced teeth and a moist handshake. The man's general appearance is suspicious of:

a. Acromegaly
b. Haemochromatosis
c. Klinefelter's syndrome
d. Gigantism
e. Hurler's syndrome

96) A 50-year-old man presents with a lump in the posterior triangle of the neck. It has been present for 8 months and is associated with a cheesy serous discharge. The most likely diagnosis is:

a. Squamous cell carcinoma
b. Tuberculous adenitis
c. Deep lobe of parotid tumour
d. Infected branchial cyst
e. Infected lymph node

97) Prophylaxis against opportunistic infections is advised when the CD4 count falls below:

a. 500 cells/mm^3
b. 300 cells/mm^3
c. 250 cells/mm^3
d. 200 cells/mm^3
e. 100 cells/mm^3

98) All the following are opportunistic infections in HIV disease EXCEPT:

   a. *Mycobacterium avium*
   b. *Toxoplasma gondii*
   c. *Pneumocystis jiroveci*
   d. Cytomegalovirus
   e. *Helicobacter pylori*

99) Recognized side effects of heparin include the following EXCEPT:

   a. Thrombocytopenic thrombosis
   b. Thrombocytopenia
   c. Alopecia
   d. Osteoporosis
   e. Hypokalaemia

100) The following statements regarding anorexia nervosa are true EXCEPT:

   a. A BMI <13 warrants hospital admission
   b. Anorexia is defined as a BMI <17.5 associated with food avoidance
   c. Physical features include bradycardia and hypotension
   d. Investigations are important in confirming the diagnosis
   e. Anorexia may be associated with reduced bone mass

101) The most useful INITIAL screening test for SLE is:

   a. Anti-dsDNA antibody
   b. Antinuclear antibody
   c. Anti-cardiolipin antibody
   d. C3 and C4 levels
   e. Anti-extractable nuclear antigen (ENA) antibody

102) Rheumatoid arthritis may be associated with all of the following EXCEPT:

   a. Ulnar drift deformity
   b. Carpal tunnel syndrome
   c. Dupuytren's contracture
   d. Painful flexor tenosynovitis
   e. Trigger finger

103) Carpal tunnel syndrome is associated with all of the following EXCEPT:

   a. Degenerative arthritis
   b. Pregnancy
   c. Acromegaly
   d. Colles' fracture
   e. Diabetes

104) A 30-year-old woman involved in an RTA is brought by ambulance to A&E. She is noted to have bruising over the mastoid process and periorbital haematoma. On otoscopic examination she has bleeding behind the tympanic membrane. The most likely diagnosis is:

   a. Extradural haematoma
   b. Subdural haematoma
   c. Basal skull fracture
   d. Depressed occipital skull fracture
   e. Intracerebral haemorrhage

105) A 54-year-old man with type 1 diabetes presents with fever, and a painful and swollen right lower leg. On examination, the pulses are absent distally, the foot is cold and subcutaneous crepitus is present. The most useful investigation is:

   a. A radiograph of the leg
   b. Doppler ultrasonography
   c. Arteriogram
   d. Blood cultures
   e. Venogram

106) The most likely diagnosis is:

   a. Osteomyelitis
   b. Gas gangrene
   c. Chronic ischaemia of the leg
   d. Deep venous thrombosis
   e. Acute ischaemia of the leg

107) A 45-year-old woman presents with pruritus, pale stools and dark urine. On examination she has finger clubbing and hepatosplenomegaly. Blood tests reveal a normal bilirubin, elevated alkaline phosphatase and low T_4. The most certain way to confirm the diagnosis is by:

   a. Anti-mitochondrial antibody
   b. Liver biopsy
   c. ERCP
   d. CT scan of the abdomen
   e. Hepatitis A, B and C serology

108) A 70-year-old man, who lives alone and is self-caring, presents with weakness in his lower legs and muscle pain. On examination he has loose teeth and is noted to have ecchymoses of the lower limbs. He suffers from rheumatoid arthritis, which greatly limits his mobility. The most likely diagnosis is:

   a. Folate deficiency
   b. Scurvy
   c. Iron deficiency
   d. Thiamine deficiency
   e. Vitamin B_{12} deficiency

109) A 20-year-old man presents with persistent eye irritation. He explains that he is sensitive to light, has noted worsening vision and complains of aching eyes. He also complains of morning stiffness in his back. The most likely diagnosis is:

   a. Keratitis
   b. Uveitis
   c. Viral conjunctivitis
   d. Episcleritis
   e. Choroiditis

110) The most useful investigation for this man would be:

   a. Lumbar and pelvic spine radiographs
   b. Kveim's test
   c. HIV test
   d. Mantoux test
   e. Rheumatoid factor

111) Which one of the following drugs CANNOT be administered via the tracheal route?

   a. Adrenaline
   b. Atropine
   c. Amiodarone
   d. Lidocaine
   e. Naloxone

112) The most specific test for SLE is:

   a. Anti-dsDNA antibody
   b. Antinuclear antibody
   c. Anti-cardiolipin antibody
   d. Rheumatoid factor
   e. Anti-extractable nuclear antigen (ENA) antibody

113) A 44-year-old woman presents with fatigue and ascites. She is noted to have a pulse of small volume. The chest radiograph is unremarkable. The 12-lead ECG shows low QRS voltage and T-wave inversion. The most likely diagnosis is:

   a. Right heart failure due to mitral stenosis
   b. Budd–Chiari syndrome
   c. Constrictive pericarditis
   d. Primary pulmonary hypertension
   e. Systemic sclerosis

114) A 38-year-old man presents with a painful right wrist and left knee joint a fortnight after an attack of gastroenteritis. Prostatic massage produces a urethral discharge. The synovial fluid shows an abundance of neutrophils and is sterile. The ESR is raised. The most likely diagnosis is:

a. Gonococcal arthritis
b. Rheumatoid arthritis
c. Salmonella arthritis
d. Reiter's syndrome
e. Viral arthritis

115) Eye signs associated with Graves' disease include all of the following EXCEPT:

a. Exophthalmos
b. Proptosis
c. External ophthalmoplegia
d. Supraorbital and infraorbital swelling
e. Ptosis

116) A 35-year-old African woman is found to have an Hb of 6 g/dL. She is a vegetarian and has a history of uterine fibroids. A blood film reveals microcytic, hypochromic red blood cells and a few target cells. The most likely diagnosis is:

a. Thalassaemia trait
b. Iron-deficiency anaemia
c. Sickle cell disease
d. Anaemia of chronic disease
e. Sideroblastic anaemia

117) A 25-year-old woman presents with a single, non-tender, enlarged, cervical lymph node. She also complains of fever and night sweats. Lymph node biopsy reveals infiltration with histiocytes and lymphocytes and the presence of cells with bilobed mirror-image nuclei. The most likely diagnosis is:

a. Non-Hodgkin's lymphoma
b. Hodgkin's lymphoma
c. Sarcoidosis
d. Acute lymphoblastic leukaemia
e. Tuberculosis

118) A 45-year-old woman with diabetes presents with shiny waxy erythematous plaques on her shins with yellowish skin and telangiectasia. The most likely diagnosis is:

a. Pretibial myxoedema
b. Pyoderma gangrenosum
c. Psoriasis
d. Erythema nodosum
e. Necrobiosis lipoidica

119) A 40-year-old man is brought to A&E in a comatose state. Useful initial investigations include all of the following EXCEPT:

a. Serum glucose
b. Serum calcium
c. Arterial blood gases
d. FBC
e. Blood alcohol level

120) On examination he is noted to have constricted pupils and depressed respirations. The most appropriate management would be:

a. CT scan of the head
b. Naloxone 0.4–1.2 mg i.v. stat
c. Flumazenil 200 mg i.v. over 15 seconds
d. Doxapram i.v.
e. Dantrolene 1 mg/kg i.v.

121) A 55-year-old man complains of generalized weakness for the past month. He also complains of excessive thirst and frequent micturition. Blood results:

Urine glucose	negative
Urine nitrate	negative
Serum creatinine	140 mmol/L
Serum urea	10 mmol/L
Serum calcium	3.5 mmol/L
Serum phosphate	1 mmol/L
Serum alkaline phosphatase	200 (30–300) IU/L
Serum albumin	45 g/L

These findings are consistent with all of the following diseases EXCEPT:

a. Primary hyperparathyroidism
b. Sarcoidosis
c. Multiple myeloma
d. Thyrotoxicosis
e. Bone metastases

122) The following are useful investigations to establish the diagnosis EXCEPT:

a. FBC
b. Chest radiograph
c. ESR
d. Parathyroid hormone
e. Magnesium

123) The chest radiograph reveals bilateral hilar lymphadenopathy. The most likely diagnosis is:

a. Multiple myeloma
b. Sarcoidosis
c. Primary hyperparathyroidism
d. Bone metastases
e. Thyrotoxicosis

124) A 30-year-old man presents with a bright red painful eye. He complains of watering of the eyes and sensitivity to light. He has a history of recurrent cold sores. Fluorescein staining of the cornea demonstrates a tree-shaped sharp-bordered stain. The most likely diagnosis is:

a. Dendritic ulcer
b. Keratoconjunctivitis sicca
c. Corneal abrasion
d. Corneal ulcer
e. Conjunctivitis

125) A 25-year-old woman presents to the outpatient clinic with a neck swelling. On examination the swelling moves upward with protrusion of the tongue. The most likely diagnosis is:

a. Thyroid goitre
b. Cystic hygroma
c. Thyroglossal cyst
d. Branchial cyst
e. Thyroid malignancy

126) A 20-year-old man arrives in A&E with marked dyspnoea; he has asthma. On examination his respiratory rate is 24/min and pulse 105/min. Peak flow is 60% of predicted. The most appropriate management would be:

a. Treat in A&E with nebulized salbutamol 5 mg and repeat peak flow in 30 min
b. Arrange immediate hospital admission and treat with intravenous hydrocortisone 200 mg
c. Arrange immediate hospital admission, administer oxygen 40–60%, nebulized salbutamol and oral prednisolone 30–60 mg
d. Arrange immediate hospital admission, administer oxygen-driven nebulizer and give slow intravenous aminophylline 250 mg
e. Treat in A&E with oral prednisolone 30–60 mg and repeat peak flow in 30 min

127) A 55-year-old man who smokes and has a history of chronic productive cough presents to A&E breathless and drowsy. On examination he is centrally cyanosed with a raised JVP (jugular venous pressure) and a palpable liver. There is a blowing pansystolic murmur at the lower left sternal border. No abnormality is heard in the lungs. The most likely diagnosis is:

   a. Infective endocarditis
   b. Cor pulmonale
   c. Rheumatic heart disease
   d. Exacerbation of chronic bronchitis
   e. Emphysema

128) The most useful investigation at this stage is:

   a. Arterial blood gas
   b. 12-lead ECG
   c. Lung function tests
   d. Chest radiograph
   e. Sputum examination

129) The most appropriate treatment is:

   a. Continuous oxygen therapy
   b. Furosemide
   c. Salbutamol inhaler
   d. Oral prednisolone 30 mg once daily
   e. Amoxicillin 500 mg three times daily

130) A 20-year-old man is found unconscious after a night of binge drinking. There is no evidence of physical trauma. On examination he has alcohol on his breath and a bitten tongue. His blood pressure is 110/80 and pulse 80/min. The pupils are small, equal and responsive to light. On removal of his clothes, his trousers are noted to be soiled with urine. The most likely suspicion is:

   a. Hypoglycaemic coma
   b. Alcohol overdose
   c. Postictal phase of an epileptic seizure
   d. Subarachnoid haemorrhage
   e. Narcotic drug overdose

131) A 42-year-old woman presents to A&E with right-sided colicky loin pain and nausea for the past 3 h. She cannot keep still because of the pain. She has a history of recurrent cystitis. Temperature 36.5°C, BP 110/60 and pulse 60/min. Urinalysis shows microscopic haematuria. The most likely diagnosis is:

   a. Pelvic inflammatory disease
   b. Acute pyelonephritis
   c. Acute appendicitis
   d. Renal colic
   e. Ectopic pregnancy

132) The most useful initial diagnostic investigation is:

   a. Serum urea and electrolytes
   b. Urine βhCG
   c. Plain KUB film
   d. Pelvic ultrasonography
   e. Intravenous urogram

133) While in A&E the patient develops fever and rigors. The most likely complication that has occurred is:

   a. Ruptured ectopic pregnancy
   b. Exacerbation of pelvic inflammatory disease
   c. Ruptured appendix
   d. Acute pyelonephritis
   e. Septicaemia

134) A 16-year-old girl is brought to A&E by her mother. She complains of persistent and worsening, dull, right-sided, lower abdominal pain and spotting of blood per vagina. The mother insists that her daughter is a virgin. On examination, her temperature is 36.5°C, BP 90/50 and pulse 120/min. The lower abdomen is rigid with rebound tenderness in the right iliac fossa. Her period is overdue. The most appropriate management following resuscitation is:

   a. To ask to speak to the girl in private, and obtain confidential information from her as to whether she has been sexually active; if so, perform urinalysis, urine βhCG pregnancy test and pelvic examination
   b. To arrange for urgent transvaginal ultrasonography to exclude ectopic pregnancy
   c. To accept that the daughter is a virgin, omit a pelvic internal examination and take a low vaginal swab to exclude infection
   d. To arrange for pelvic ultrasonography to exclude ectopic pregnancy and acute appendicitis.
   e. To inform the mother that you are performing a urine pregnancy test in the best interests of her daughter to exclude the possibility of a miscarriage or ectopic pregnancy

135) The most appropriate treatment for a dendritic ulcer of the eye is:

   a. Prednisolone 0.5% 6 hourly
   b. Aciclovir 3% eye ointment five times daily
   c. Chloramphenicol 1% eye ointment
   d. Aciclovir 800 mg five times daily
   e. Cefuroxime 50 mg/mL

136) A 40-year-old woman presents with dysuria and urinary incontinence. She has a history of having passed urinary calculi in the past. The urine is noted to have an alkaline pH. The most likely organism is:

a. *Escherichia coli*
b. *Proteus mirabilis*
c. Atypical streptococci
d. *Pseudomonas aeruginosa*
e. *Klebsiella* sp.

137) A 40-year-old pedestrian has been struck by a speeding car. He is brought to A&E wearing a pneumatic anti-shock garment for an extensive, open, avulsion injury to his pelvis. He is intubated with fluids running via two large-bore intravenous cannulas. His blood pressure is 120/80. The pelvis is grossly distorted. The next most appropriate management would be to:

a. Take blood for FBC, type and crossmatch 6 units, urea and electrolytes, and start O-negative blood infusion
b. Cut away the man's clothing and perform a thorough physical examination
c. Insert a Foley catheter after a digital rectal examination to exclude a high-riding prostate
d. Perform a brief neurological examination
e. Notify the orthopaedic surgeons to apply an external fixator

138) An 18-year-old young man presents with fever, stridor and trismus. His breathing becomes laboured with use of accessory muscles. He becomes cyanosed with a respiratory rate of 35, despite oxygen by facemask. He had initially presented to his GP a few days ago with a sore throat. He uses a salbutamol inhaler for his asthma. The most appropriate management in A&E would be:

a. Endotracheal intubation
b. Needle cricothyroidotomy
c. Tracheostomy
d. Intravenous hydrocortisone
e. Nasopharyngeal airway

139) The most likely diagnosis is:

a. Glandular fever
b. Streptococcal throat infection
c. Acute asthma attack
d. Angioneurotic oedema
e. Tetanus

140) A 60-year-old woman presents with progressive forgetfulness and mood changes. She has a shuffling gait. Her brain CT scan shows cortical atrophy and enlarged ventricles. Histology shows senile plaques and neurofibrillary tangles. The most appropriate treatment is:

   a. Levodopa in combination with a dopa-decarboxylase inhibitor
   b. Donepezil
   c. Tetrabenazine
   d. Diazepam
   e. Thiamine

141) Charcot's joints are a recognized feature of all the following conditions EXCEPT:

   a. Leprosy
   b. Diabetes mellitus
   c. Syringomyelia
   d. Syphilis
   e. Rheumatoid arthritis

142) A 60-year-old priest presents with cough, dyspnoea, dull chest pain and vague epigastric pain. On examination the left chest shows diminished expansion, stony dull percussion note and absent breath sounds. There is egophony at the apex. The mediastinum is shifted to the right. The chest radiograph confirms a unilateral pleural effusion. The most useful investigation would be:

   a. CT of the chest
   b. Sputum for culture and sensitivity
   c. Aspiration of pleural effusion
   d. Bronchoscopy
   e. Ventilation—perfusion scan

143) A 60-year-old man presents with increasing abdominal girth. On examination you elicit shifting dullness. The most useful investigation would be:

   a. CT scan of the abdomen
   b. Ascitic fluid tap
   c. Ultrasonography of the abdomen
   d. Chest radiograph
   e. Blood for FBC, U&Es, LFTs and amylase

144) A 45-year-old woman presents with severe itching, recent pale stools and dark urine. On examination there is darkened skin pigmentation, xanthelasma and hepatomegaly. Test results are as follows:

Serum bilirubin	15 mmol/L
Serum alkaline phosphatase	400 (30–300) IU/L
AST	40 (5–35) IU/L

The most likely diagnosis is:

a. Sarcoidosis
b. Primary biliary cirrhosis
c. Sclerosing cholangitis
d. Acute cholecystitis
e. Common bile duct gallstones

145) *Neisseria gonorrhoeae* may infect all of the following areas EXCEPT the:

a. Vagina
b. Rectum
c. Pharynx
d. Conjunctiva
e. Urethra

146) A 30-year-old woman with Crohn's disease presents with left flank pain and microscopic haematuria. She admits that she doesn't drink enough water. She smokes, drinks wine and loves chocolates. A radiograph shows a radio-opaque left renal calculus. The most likely aetiology is:

a. Hypercalciuria
b. Hyperoxaluria
c. Hyperuricaemia
d. Cystinuria
e. Hyperuricosuria

147) Dietary recommendations that you would make for her include avoidance of all of the following EXCEPT:

a. Spinach
b. Rhubarb
c. Chocolate
d. Tomatoes
e. Tea

148) A 50-year-old man with known liver disease presents with fever, abdominal pain and distension. On examination he has a tender abdomen with shifting dullness. Diagnostic aspiration shows elevated neutrophils. Gram stain shows Gram-negative rods. The most likely organism is:

    a. *Klebsiella* sp.
    b. *Escherichia coli*
    c. *Pseudomonas aeruginosa*
    d. *Bacteroides fragilis*
    e. *Streptococcus pneumoniae*

149) Causes of air under the diaphragm include all of the following EXCEPT:

    a. Crohn's disease
    b. Perforated duodenal ulcer
    c. Pleuroperitoneal fistula
    d. Laparoscopy
    e. Ruptured ectopic pregnancy

150) A 30-year-old man presents with fever, arthralgia and a palmar rash. On examination he has oral vesicles and target-like lesions on his palms. The most likely diagnosis is:

    a. Stevens–Johnson syndrome
    b. Behçet's syndrome
    c. Herpes simplex
    d. Syphilis
    e. Hand–foot–mouth disease

151) A 50-year-old man presents in shock with rigors and a temperature of 40°C. He is jaundiced and tender on palpation of the liver, which is felt 5 cm below the costal margin. Dark concentrated urine is noted on Foley catheter insertion. The most likely diagnosis is:

    a. Ascending cholangitis
    b. Gallstone ileus
    c. Hepatitis
    d. Primary sclerosing cholangitis
    e. Acute cholecystitis

152) A 60-year-old woman presents with morning stiffness in both knees and pain worse at the end of the day. On examination the knees are swollen and warm to the touch. She has a flexion deformity and limitation of movement. A radiograph shows narrowing of the joint spaces, osteophytes at the margin of the joints and sclerosis of the underlying bone. The most likely diagnosis is:

    a. Rheumatoid arthritis
    b. Osteoarthritis
    c. Gout
    d. Infective arthritis
    e. Polymyalgia rheumatica

153) Recognized treatments for this condition include all of the following EXCEPT:

a. Total knee replacement
b. NSAIDs
c. Penicillamine
d. Intra-articular corticosteroid
e. Physiotherapy

154) A 70-year-old man presents with progressive stepwise dementia associated with focal neurological events. He has a stiff, slow-moving, spastic tongue, dysarthria, and inappropriate laughing and crying. He walks with a shuffling gait taking small steps. He is also noted to be hypertensive. The most likely diagnosis is:

a. Parkinson's disease
b. Alzheimer's disease
c. Multi-infarct dementia
d. Lateral medullary syndrome
e. Multiple sclerosis

155) A 20-year-old man complains of recurrent lower back pain and stiffness after exercise. He has no morning stiffness. Full blood count and ESR are normal, but he is found to have HLA B27. Radiographs of his lumbar spine and pelvis are normal. The most appropriate management would be:

a. No further investigations and reassure that HLA B27 can also be found normally
b. Arrange for an ophthalmology referral for slit-lamp examination
c. Arrange Kveim's test to exclude sarcoidosis
d. Arrange for barium follow-through
e. Test for rheumatoid factor

156) A 55-year-old man with type 1 diabetes presents with nausea, lethargy, and dry and itchy yellow–brown skin. He also complains of nocturia and impotence. His blood film shows normocytic normochromic anaemia and occasional Burr cells. The most appropriate management would be:

a. Start iron replacement therapy
b. Take blood for U&Es
c. Check HbA1c
d. Take blood for bilirubin, LFTs and amylase
e. Take blood for thyroid function tests

157) Cystic fibrosis is associated with all of the following EXCEPT:

a. Abnormal gene coding for transmembrane regulating factor protein on chromosome 7
b. Allergic bronchopulmonary aspergillosis
c. Steatorrhoea
d. Chronic infection with *Pseudomonas pseudomallei*
e. Diabetes mellitus

158) A 20-year-old pregnant black woman presents with fever and joint pains. She has a history of two previous spontaneous early miscarriages. Urine reveals ++ protein. Blood results show leucopenia, normocytic normochromic anaemia and thrombocytopenia. The most likely diagnosis is:

   a. Sickle cell disease
   b. SLE
   c. Thalassaemia
   d. Aplastic anaemia
   e. Pre-eclampsia

159) The most sensitive diagnostic test would be:

   a. A PET screen
   b. Antibodies to dsDNA
   c. Positive antinuclear antibodies
   d. Antibody to Ro
   e. Haemoglobin electrophoresis

160) The most useful investigation for her miscarriages would be:

   a. Transvaginal ultrasonography
   b. Chromosome karyotype
   c. Lupus anticoagulant and anticardiolipin antibody
   d. Hysterosalpingogram
   e. Antithrombin III, and protein C and S deficiency

161) The most common organism implicated in acute bacterial endocarditis is:

   a. *Staphylococcus aureus*
   b. *Streptococcus viridans*
   c. *Streptococcus faecalis*
   d. *Staphylococcus epidermidis*
   e. *Coxiella burnetii*

162) A 25-year-old heroin addict presents with fever and mucosal petechial haemorrhages. On examination he has a pansystolic murmur best heard at the lower sternal edge. He is also noted to have small, flat, erythematous, non-tender macules over the thenar eminence. The most likely diagnosis is:

   a. Subacute bacterial endocarditis
   b. Acute bacterial endocarditis
   c. Rheumatic heart disease
   d. Acute rheumatic fever
   e. Q fever

163) Major criteria for the diagnosis of rheumatic fever include all of the following EXCEPT:

    a. Polyarthralgia
    b. Chorea
    c. Erythema marginatum
    d. Subcutaneous nodules
    e. Fever

164) The organism responsible for gas gangrene is:

    a. *Clostridium difficile*
    b. *Clostridium perfringens*
    c. *Clostridium tetani*
    d. *Klebsiella* sp.
    e. *Pseudomonas aeruginosa*

165) Which one of the following features would favour a diagnosis of Guillain–Barré syndrome rather than myasthenia gravis?

    a. Ocular muscle involvement
    b. Proximal muscle weakness
    c. Respiratory difficulties
    d. Areflexia
    e. Facial muscle weakness

166) The most common cause of painless frank haematuria in male patients aged over 50 years is:

    a. Bladder squamous cell carcinoma
    b. Carcinoma of the prostate
    c. Hypernephroma
    d. Transitional cell carcinoma in the kidney
    e. Transitional cell bladder carcinoma

167) A 30-year-old man presents to A&E with a tender swollen testicle. He states that he was struck in the groin while playing football. On examination the borders of the testicle are irregular, and the testicle is heavy and woody. There is no associated lymphadenopathy. He is also noted to have gynaecomastia. There are no external signs of trauma. The most appropriate initial management would be:

    a. Take blood for α-fetoprotein and βhCG and arrange for a chest radiograph
    b. Prescribe doxycycline 100 mg twice daily for 5 days
    c. Refer to urologist for urgent surgical exploration
    d. Arrange for a chest and abdominal CT scan
    e. Arrange for ultrasonography of the testes

168) A 20-year-old woman presents with acne and hirsutism. She complains of a year of chaotic menstrual cycles with long periods of amenorrhoea. She has gained weight recently. She has never been pregnant. On examination there are no other abnormalities. The most likely diagnosis is:

a. Congenital adrenal hyperplasia
b. Ovarian teratoma
c. Cushing's disease
d. Testicular feminization
e. Polycystic ovarian disease

169) Treatment for multiple sclerosis includes all of the following EXCEPT:

a. Glatiramer actetate
b. Interferon-β1a
c. Interferon-β1b
d. Interferon-α
e. Baclofen

170) The following features would favour a diagnosis of ulcerative colitis rather than Crohn's disease:

a. Uveitis
b. Arthritis
c. Pyoderma gangrenosum
d. Cholelithiasis
e. Pseudopolyps

171) A 50-year-old man presents with polydipsia, headache and weakness. On examination his BP is 160/100 but he is not oedematous. He takes no medication. Blood results reveal hypokalaemia, alkalosis and low serum renin. The most likely diagnosis is:

a. Conn's syndrome
b. Secondary hyperaldosteronism
c. Cushing's disease
d. Phaeochromocytoma
e. Renal artery stenosis

172) A 25-year-old healthy man who smokes presents with gangrene of the left big toe. There are no signs of external trauma. The most likely diagnosis is:

a. Thrombangiitis obliterans (Buerger's disease)
b. Raynaud's disease
c. Gas gangrene
d. Polyarteritis nodosa
e. Gout

173) Peptic ulcer disease is associated with all of the following EXCEPT:

    a. Head trauma
    b. Burns
    c. Chronic pancreatitis
    d. Hypocalcaemia
    e. Cirrhosis

174) The most common cause of massive upper gastrointestinal bleeding is:

    a. Gastric ulcer
    b. Duodenal ulcer
    c. Oesophageal varices
    d. Mallory–Weiss syndrome
    e. Angiodysplasia

175) A 35-year-old African woman is found to have a Hb of 6 g/dL. She is a vegetarian and has a history of uterine fibroids. Blood film reveals microcytic hypochromic red blood cells and a few target cells. The most likely result of iron studies would be:

    a. Low ferritin, high total iron-binding capacity (TIBC)
    b. Low iron, low TIBC
    c. Raised ferritin, low TIBC
    d. Low serum iron, low TIBC
    e. Normal ferritin, high TIBC

176) A 40-year-old long-stay patient in a psychiatric hospital presents with fever, abdominal pain, dry cough and worsening confusion. Blood tests reveal neutrophilia, lymphopenia and hyponatraemia. A chest radiograph shows right-sided lobar consolidation. The most appropriate treatment would be:

    a. Erythromycin
    b. Benzylpenicillin
    c. Antituberculous chemotherapy
    d. Ciprofloxacin
    e. Ticarcillin

177) Diseases associated with impotence include all of the following EXCEPT:

    a. Hyperthyroidism
    b. Hyperprolactinaemia
    c. Cirrhosis
    d. Multiple sclerosis
    e. Renal failure

178) The following organisms and disease are correctly paired EXCEPT:

a. β-haemolytic streptococci – necrotizing fasciitis
b. *Staphylococcus epidermis* – toxic shock syndrome
c. *Staphylococcus aureus* – scalded skin syndrome
d. *S. aureus* – impetigo
e. Group A β-haemolytic streptococci – acute rheumatic fever

179) A 20-year-old man who has travelled recently to India presents with unexplained fever for 5 days. You suspect typhoid fever. The most appropriate investigation would be:

a. Widal's test measuring serum levels of agglutinins to O and H antigens
b. Blood culture
c. Marrow culture
d. Stool culture
e. Urine culture

180) The following statements regarding sarcoidosis are correct EXCEPT:

a. There is a higher incidence among young black males than white individuals
b. It most commonly involves the mediastinal lymph nodes
c. A third of cases are associated with erythema nodosum
d. Scalene node biopsy will be positive in 90% of cases
e. A negative Kveim test excludes sarcoidosis.

181) A 70-year-old man presents with chronic cough, haemoptysis and weight loss. He smokes 20 cigarettes a day. A chest radiograph shows a central coin lesion. The most useful investigation would be:

a. Sputum for culture and cytology
b. Isotope bone scan
c. Bronchoscopy and biopsy
d. Percutaneous needle biopsy
e. CT scan of the chest

182) A 70-year-old woman presents with vertigo when rolling over in bed. She also notices that she gets dizzy when bending over or reaching for the top shelf. The cause of her vertigo is:

a. Migraine
b. Benign positional vertigo
c. Acoustic neuroma
d. Ménière's disease
e. Acute vestibular neuronitis

183) The most common viral illness in transplant recipients is:

   a. HIV
   b. Herpes zoster
   c. Herpes simplex
   d. CMV
   e. Epstein–Barr virus

184) A 30-year-old woman presents with a diffusely enlarged thyroid gland associated with a bruit. Serum thyroxine is raised and TSH is low. The most discriminating investigation would be:

   a. Ultrasound scan
   b. Fine-needle biopsy
   c. Serum thyroid-stimulating immunoglobulins against TSH receptor
   d. Radioiodine scan
   e. Thyroid-releasing hormone (TRH) test

185) A 50-year-old woman is noted to have a high serum calcium, low–normal phosphate and normal albumin on routine biochemistry test. She is asymptomatic. The most useful additional blood test would be:

   a. Serum chloride
   b. Serum parathyroid hormone (PTH)
   c. Serum magnesium
   d. Serum urea
   e. Serum alkaline phosphatase

186) The serum PTH comes back as high. The most useful investigation to confirm the diagnosis is:

   a. Skull radiograph
   b. Pelvic radiograph
   c. Radioisotope thallium/technetium subtraction scan of the neck
   d. Chest radiograph
   e. CT scan of the neck

187) A 90-year-old man is noted to have a serum alkaline phosphatase of 1050 (30–300) IU/L on routine blood tests. He is asymptomatic. Serum calcium, phosphate and PTH levels are normal. The most likely diagnosis is:

   a. Multiple myeloma
   b. Paget's disease (osteitis deformans)
   c. Bone metastases
   d. Hyperparathyroidism
   e. Osteomalacia

188) A 20-year-old man back from hitchhiking through South America a fortnight ago now presents with explosive, watery, foul-smelling diarrhoea and weight loss. On examination he has abdominal distension. His stools are greasy and contain mucus. The most useful investigation would be:

a. Proctoscopy
b. Sodium sweat test
c. Abdominal radiograph
d. Stool for microscopy
e. Duodenal aspirate

189) A 60-year-old man postgastrectomy presents with macrocystic anaemia. He drinks alcohol regularly. The most likely cause of his anaemia is:

a. Coeliac disease
b. Pernicious anaemia
c. Iron deficiency
d. Vitamin B_{12} deficiency
e. Thalassaemia

190) A 30-year-old man presents in a coma after a drug overdose. His pupils are dilated, and he is hypotensive. His pulse rate drops to 40 and ECG confirms second-degree Mobitz type II heart block. The most likely cause of his overdose is:

a. Barbiturate
b. Tricyclic antidepressant
c. Lithium
d. β blocker
e. Benzodiazepine

191) A 50-year-old obese man presents with headache and drowsiness. He has a history of snoring. He has warm extremities, a flapping tremor and a bounding pulse. The most likely cause for these symptoms is:

a. CO_2 retention
b. Hypoxia
c. Obstructive sleep apnoea
d. Cerebral tumour
e. Malignant hypertension

192) A 25-year-old woman presents to A&E with light-headedness and breathlessness. She complains of tingling and numbness of her hands. Arterial blood gases:

pH	7.55
Pa_{CO_2}	3 kPa
Pa_{O_2}	14 kPa
H^+	25 nmol/L
HCO_3^-	20 mmol/L

The most appropriate management would be:

a. Chest radiograph
b. Breathe into a paper bag
c. Activated charcoal
d. Needle thoracocentesis
e. $\dot{V}/\dot{Q}$ scan

193) A 20-year-old man with asthma presents with increased shortness of breath. On chest examination he is found to have a deviated trachea to the right, reduced tactile fremitus and hyperresonance to percussion on the left. The most likely diagnosis is:

a. Right-sided pulmonary embolism
b. Right-sided pneumothorax
c. Left-sided pneumothorax
d. Left bronchopneumonia
e. Left-sided pleural effusion

194) A 50-year-old man presents with weight loss, hiccoughs, jaundice, epigastric and right upper quadrant pain radiating to the back. On examination he is noted to have hepatomegaly, a palpable gallbladder, and an abdominal bruit heard in the periumbilical area and left upper quadrant. The most likely diagnosis is:

a. Abdominal aortic aneurysm
b. Gallbladder carcinoma
c. Hepatocellular carcinoma
d. Carcinoma of the head of the pancreas
e. Cholecystitis

195) Recognized side effects of thiazide diuretics include all of the following EXCEPT:

a. Hyperuricaemia
b. Increased LDL-cholesterol
c. Hypokalaemia
d. Hypoglycaemia
e. Hypercalcaemia

196) First-line therapy for hypertension in a pregnant woman is:
   a. Labetalol
   b. Hydralazine
   c. Methyldopa
   d. Bendrofluazide
   e. Nifedipine

197) A 50-year-old man with type 1 diabetes presents with peripheral oedema and ascites. He has +++ proteinuria. A 24-hour urine collection contains 10 g protein. Serum albumin is 15 g/L. The most likely diagnosis is:
   a. Diabetic nephrosclerosis
   b. Nephrotic syndrome
   c. Uraemia
   d. Interstitial nephritis
   e. Retroperitoneal fibrosis

198) A 25-year-old HIV-positive man presents with 2 weeks of worsening drowsiness. On examination he has cervical lymphadenopathy and has bilateral upgoing plantar reflexes. A CT scan of the head shows cerebral calcifications and ring lesions. The most likely diagnosis is:
   a. Cerebral toxoplasmosis
   b. Cerebral abscess
   c. Lymphoma
   d. Cryptococcal meningitis
   e. Tuberculosis

199) A 12-year-old boy presents to A&E with severe dyspnoea. He had been treated by his GP with penicillin for presumed tonsillitis. He uses a salbutamol inhaler for asthma. On examination: temperature 40°C and he is drooling saliva; no trismus. Marked inspiratory stridor and a respiratory rate of 30/min. The most appropriate management would be:
   a. Oxygen-driven nebulizer
   b. Intravenous hydrocortisone
   c. Indirect laryngoscopy
   d. Endotracheal intubation under general anaesthesia
   e. Cricothyroidotomy

200) The most likely diagnosis is:
   a. Croup
   b. Acute epiglottitis
   c. Glandular fever
   d. Acute streptococcal tonsillitis
   e. Acute severe asthma attack

201) A 50-year-old man with a history of previous myocardial infarction presents to A&E with chest pain. The initial blood pressure is 110/70. During evaluation, he collapses. ECG shows ventricular tachycardia. He has no palpable pulse. The most appropriate management would be:

a. Synchronized DC shock at 100 J
b. Administer amiodarone 150 mg i.v. over 10 min
c. DC cardioversion with 200 J
d. Administer lidocaine 50 mg i.v. over 2 min
e. Commence CPR (cardiopulmonary resuscitation)

202) An 80-year-old woman presents with chronic dysphagia and weight loss. She complains of a sensation of a lump in her throat, bad breath and regurgitation of undigested food. She has a history of recurrent chest infections. She does not smoke or drink alcohol. Physical examination reveals a low BMI and a visible lump on the left side of her neck, which is difficult to define on palpation. The best initial investigation would be:

a. Chest radiograph
b. Barium meal
c. Endoscopy and biopsy
d. Oesophageal motility studies
e. Indirect laryngoscopy

203) A 30-year-old woman presents with bilateral ptosis and diplopia. She has also noticed difficulty in swallowing. The most likely diagnosis is:

a. Dystrophia myotonica
b. Multiple sclerosis
c. Polymyositis
d. Myasthenic syndrome (Eaton–Lambert syndrome)
e. Myasthenia gravis

204) A 20-year-old woman presents with complete right ptosis. On lifting the eyelid, the eye is seen to be looking down and out. The pupil is dilated. The most likely diagnosis is:

a. Right third nerve and right superior oblique palsy
b. Complete right third nerve palsy
c. Incomplete right third nerve palsy
d. Horner's syndrome
e. Right third nerve and lateral rectus palsy

205) The organism most frequently isolated from the ascitic fluid of patients with spontaneous bacterial peritonitis is:

a. *Klebsiella* sp
b. *Escherichia coli*
c. *Streptococcus pneumoniae*
d. *Bacteroides fragilis*
e. *Pseudomonas aeruginosa*

206) A 40-year-old man with a prosthetic heart valve on warfarin anticoagulation presents with haematuria. His INR is 4. The most appropriate management after withholding warfarin would be:

a. Give 0.5–2 mg of vitamin K by slow intravenous injection
b. No further treatment and recheck INR in 1–2 days
c. Commence heparin
d. Give 1 L of FFP (fresh frozen plasma)
e. Give prothrombin complex concentrate (factor 9A) and factor VII

207) A 22-year-old woman presents with secondary amenorrhoea and weight loss. On examination she is noted to have mild parotid swelling. She has a low BP and a BMI of 15. The most likely reason for her amenorrhoea is:

a. Prolactinoma
b. Addison's disease
c. Premature ovarian failure
d. Anorexia nervosa
e. Bulimia

208) The inspired oxygen content using a bag–valve–mask with oxygen but no reservoir is:

a. 16%
b. 21%
c. 40%
d. 50%
e. 80%

209) The most common cause of new-onset focal or generalized seizures after the age of 50 is:

a. Alcoholism
b. Brain abscess
c. Brain tumour
d. Cerebrovascular disease
e. Encephalitis

210) A 50 year old presents with weight loss, increased appetite, sweating, palpitations, tremors and preference for cold weather. The most useful diagnostic investigation is:

a. Chest radiograph
b. Serum glucose
c. U&Es
d. TFTs
e. FBC

211) A 15-year-old boy presents with high swinging fever and arthritis affecting the knees. The joints are swollen but not very tender. Blood tests reveal anaemia and a raised ESR. Rheumatoid factor is negative but ANAs are positive. The most likely diagnosis is:

a. Acute rheumatic fever
b. Juvenile rheumatoid arthritis
c. Still's disease
d. Osteochondritis dissecans
e. Aseptic non-traumatic synovitis

212) The next most appropriate step to guide your further management would be:

a. Echocardiography
b. Aspiration of knee joint
c. Arrange for MRI of the knee
d. Arrange for ophthalmology referral for slit-lamp examination
e. Blood cultures

213) A 30-year-old man presents with acute loin pain and haematuria. He has a history of recurrent urinary tract infections. He states that his father also had kidney problems and had suffered from a bleed in the brain. On examination his BP is 160/100, and he has ballotable, large, irregular kidneys and hepatomegaly. The most definitive investigation would be:

a. Kidney–ureter–bladder (KUB) plain film
b. Excretion urography
c. CT scan of the abdomen
d. Renal ultrasonography
e. Urinalysis and MSU for culture and sensitivities

214) The inspired oxygen content using a bag–valve–mask with oxygen and reservoir is:

a. 16%
b. 21%
c. 40%
d. 50%
e. 80%

215) Postsplenectomy complications include all of the following EXCEPT:

a. Increased susceptibility to falciparum malaria infection
b. Increased susceptibility to *Haemophilus influenzae* infection
c. Pneumococcal septicaemia
d. Thromboembolism
e. Thrombocytopenia

216) A 60-year-old man with a history of angina presents with chest pain. ECG shows ventricular tachycardia. Pulse rate is 200/min and BP 80/50. Oxygen is applied by facemask. Initial management should be:

a. Administer sedation and call urgently for the anaesthetist
b. Immediate synchronized cardioversion at 100 J
c. Immediate unsynchronized DC cardioversion at 200 J
d. Adenosine i.v.
e. Lidocaine i.v.

217) A 20-year-old man complains of high fever, rigors, productive cough with rusty-coloured sputum and pleuritic chest pain. On chest examination he has increased tactile fremitus and dullness to percussion in the right lower lung field. The most likely diagnosis is:

a. Lobar pneumonia
b. Bronchopneumonia
c. Aspiration pneumonia
d. Pleural effusion
e. Lung abscess

218) A 40-year-old woman presents with multiple symptoms. She states that for weeks she has felt tired with a loss of appetite. She has intermittent abdominal pain and diarrhoea, and has lost half a stone in weight. On examination: temperature 36.5°C, supine BP 100/60 with a pulse of 90/min, postural hypotension, mild epigastric pain and a pigmented appendectomy scar. The most likely diagnosis is:

a. Hypopituitarism
b. Diabetes mellitus
c. Addison's disease
d. Hyperthyroidism
e. Crohn's syndrome

219) A 25-year-old obese woman presents with mood swings, acne, secondary amenorrhoea and hirsutism. She has mild lower back pain, which she relates to her weight problem. She smokes 20 cigarettes a day and drinks alcohol on the weekends. Her BP is 125/85 and urine dipstick is negative for glucose. The most likely diagnosis is:

a. Cushing's syndrome
b. Polycystic ovary syndrome
c. Congenital adrenal hyperplasia
d. Ovarian carcinoma
e. Hypothyroidism

220) A 90-year-old man is noted to have a serum alkaline phosphatase of 1050 (30–300) IU/L on routine blood tests. He is asymptomatic. Serum calcium, phosphate and PTH levels are normal. The most appropriate treatment would be:

   a. Nil
   b. Parathyroid surgeon referral
   c. Chest radiograph
   d. Vitamin D therapy
   e. Calcitonin

221) A 50-year-old obese man is brought to A&E in a confused state. On examination he has nystagmus and is unable to move the eyes fully laterally. He walks with a broad-based gait. He is unaware of his surroundings and grows restless. The most likely diagnosis is:

   a. Subdural haematoma
   b. Creutzfeldt–Jakob syndrome
   c. Wernicke's encephalopathy
   d. Korsakoff's psychosis
   e. Hypoglycaemia

222) A 60-year-old woman with rheumatoid arthritis presents with numbness and tingling in the thumb and first two fingers of the right hand. It is worse at night. On examination there is sensory loss in the right hand involving the lateral half of the ring finger and dorsal tips of the first two fingers. The patient is able to flex the interphalangeal joint of the index finger on clasping the hands (Oschner's test). The most likely diagnosis is:

   a. Complete median nerve lesion
   b. Carpal tunnel syndrome
   c. Median and ulnar nerve palsy
   d. Cervical spondylosis
   e. Cervical rib

223) The most useful investigation is:

   a. Wrist radiograph
   b. MRI of the neck
   c. Nerve conduction studies
   d. Hand radiograph
   e. Chest radiograph

224) A 40-year-old man presents with diplopia and pain over the left eye. His medication includes lisinopril and Humulin insulin. On examination he has an almost total ophthalmoplegia with sparing of lateral eye movement on the left. His pupils are symmetrical, reactive to light, and of normal size and shape. The most likely diagnosis is:

   a. Nerve III palsy due to compression
   b. Mononeuritis involving nerve III
   c. Complete nerve III palsy
   d. Argyll Robertson pupil
   e. Myasthenia gravis

225) A 30-year-old woman presents with severe headache and vomiting. She is sensitive to light and also complains of neck pain. Her BP is 170/110 and pulse 50. On examination she has bilateral ptosis and dilated pupils, and her eyes are positioned down and out. On fundoscopic examination bilateral papilloedema is present. Protein and glucose are present in her urine. Her mental status deteriorates rapidly. The most likely diagnosis is:

   a. Intracranial tumour
   b. Subdural haematoma
   c. Subarachnoid haemorrhage
   d. Extradural haematoma
   e. Intracerebral haemorrhage

226) The most appropriate investigation is:

   a. Lumbar puncture
   b. CT scan of the head
   c. MRI of the brain
   d. Cerebral angiography
   e. EEG

227) A 50-year-old woman complains of episodes of diplopia and vertigo, worse after exercise. On examination the BP in her right arm is 120/80 and in her left arm 100/60. A cervical bruit is noted. The most likely diagnosis is:

   a. Coarctation of the aorta
   b. Transient ischaemic attack
   c. Takayasu's arteritis
   d. Subclavian steal syndrome
   e. Vertebrobasilar insufficiency

228) A 50-year-old obese man presents with headache and drowsiness. He has a history of snoring. He has warm extremities, a flapping tremor and a bounding pulse. On fundoscopic examination papilloedema is present. The most appropriate treatment would be:

a. Flumazenil
b. Doxapram
c. Naloxone
d. Hyperbaric oxygen
e. Diazepam

229) A 70-year-old man presents with nausea, vomiting and weakness. He has marked peripheral oedema. His medications include digoxin and chlorthalidone for congestive heart failure. Furosemide is administered to which he has marked diuresis of 10 L and promptly collapses. ECG shows prolonged P–R interval, inverted T waves and depressed ST segments. The most useful blood test is:

a. CK-MB and troponin
b. Serum U&Es
c. Digoxin level
d. Serum osmolality
e. Random cortisol

230) A 40-year-old man presents with painful, asymmetrical, deforming arthritis involving the distal interphalangeal joints and lower back pain. His fingernails are pitted with onycholysis. The most likely diagnosis is:

a. Rheumatoid arthritis
b. Ankylosing spondylitis
c. Psoriatic arthritis
d. Osteoarthritis
e. Ulcerative colitis

231) A 16-year-old boy presents with gynaecomastia. On examination his arm span exceeds the body length and he has small, firm testes. The most likely diagnosis is:

a. Testicular feminization
b. Congenital adrenal hyperplasia
c. Klinefelter's syndrome
d. True hermaphroditism
e. Adrenal 5α-reductase deficiency

232) A 45-year-old woman who underwent mastectomy with axillary clearance 2 years ago now presents with excessive thirst and polyuria. Investigations show:

Serum sodium	150 mmol/L
Serum potassium	3.8 mmol/L
Serum calcium	2.8 mmol/L
Random serum glucose	9 mmol/L
Serum urea	6 mmol/L
Serum creatinine	100 mmol/L
Urine osmolality	150 mosmol/L

The most likely diagnosis is:

a. Psychogenic polydipsia
b. SIADH
c. Diabetes insipidus
d. Hypercalcaemia
e. Diabetes mellitus

233) A 65-year-old woman presents to A&E with breathlessness and chest pain. On examination the pulse is irregularly irregular and ECG confirms atrial fibrillation at a rate of 180/min. You administer oxygen and gain intravenous access. The next most appropriate step in management would be:

a. Heparin and warfarin anticoagulation
b. Immediate heparin and synchronized DC shock at 100 J
c. Amiodarone 300 mg i.v. over 1 h
d. Intravenous digoxin
e. Flecainide 100 mg i.v. over 30 min

234) A 60-year-old man presents with rigidity and bradykinesia. He has an ataxic gait. On examination he has postural hypotension without compensatory tachycardia and his pupils are asymmetrical.

a. Multi-infarct dementia
b. Alzheimer's disease
c. Friedrich's ataxia
d. Parkinson's disease
e. Multi-system atrophy (MSA)

235) An 80-year-old woman presents with chronic dysphagia and weight loss. She complains of a sensation of a lump in her throat, bad breath and regurgitation of undigested food. She has a history of recurrent chest infections. She does not smoke or drink alcohol. Physical examination reveals a low BMI and a visible lump on the left side of her neck, which is difficult to define on palpation. The most likely diagnosis is:

a. Squamous cell carcinoma of the oesophagus
b. Pharyngeal pouch
c. Achalasia
d. Cricopharyngeal spasm
e. Postcricoid carcinoma

236) A 60-year-old woman presents with sudden painless loss of vision in her right eye. There is no perception of light and there is an afferent pupillary defect. The retina is white with a cherry-red spot at the macula. The optic discs are swollen. She also has a right-sided carotid bruit. The most likely diagnosis is:

a. Retinal detachment
b. Optic neuritis
c. Central retinal vein occlusion
d. Ischaemic optic neuropathy
e. Central retinal artery occlusion

237) A 20-year-old woman presents with fatigue, nausea, vomiting and abdominal colic. She has been feeling unwell for many months now and lives as a squatter in a derelict old house. On examination she is noted to have signs of peripheral neuropathy with a wrist drop. Blood film shows basophilic stippling of red blood cells. The most likely diagnosis is:

a. Thalassaemia
b. Iron poisoning
c. Lead poisoning
d. Crohn's disease
e. Carbon monoxide poisoning

238) A 28-year-old Jamaican woman presents with acute onset of nausea, vomiting, epigastric pain and ascites. She does not take any medication apart from traditional herbal remedies. On examination she has tender hepatomegaly and profound ascites but no signs of heart failure. She has abnormal LFTs. The ascitic fluid has high protein content. The investigation of choice is:

a. Isotope scanning of the liver
b. Hepatic venography
c. Liver biopsy
d. Ultrasound scan
e. Abdominal radiograph

239) The most likely diagnosis is:

a. Primary biliary cirrhosis
b. Hepatic vein thrombosis
c. Alcoholic hepatitis
d. Portal vein thrombosis
e. Meigs' syndrome

240) A 30-year-old HIV-positive man presents with seizures. The most likely infective cause is:

a. Toxoplasmosis
b. Cytomegalovirus
c. *Cryptosporidium* sp.
d. Tuberculosis
e. Pneumocystosis

241) Which of the following illicit drugs is still detectable in urine up to a month later?

a. Cocaine
b. Cannabis
c. Methadone
d. Heroin
e. Amphetamine

242) The following are recognized features of obstructive sleep apnoea EXCEPT:

a. Hypnagogic hallucinations
b. Impotence
c. Morning headaches
d. Nightmares
e. Daydreaming

243) A 50-year-old woman presents to medical outpatients complaining of pain and stiffness in the joints of her hands, worse in the mornings. The pain lasts for a couple of hours in the morning. On examination she has ulnar deviation, wasting of the small muscles of her hands, nail pitting and a rash on her knees. There is symmetrical involvement of the distal interphalangeal joints and metacarpophalangeal joints. The most likely diagnosis is:

a. Rheumatoid arthritis
b. Psoriatic arthropathy
c. Sjögren's syndrome
d. SLE
e. Osteoarthritis

244) A 70-year-old man presents to A&E after falling when drunk. He complains of sudden numbness and tingling all over both his legs. He also complains of pain between the shoulder blades. On examination he has weakness in his lower extremities, hyperreflexia, positive Babinski's sign and clonus. The most likely diagnosis is:

a. Motor neuron disease
b. Subacute combined degeneration of the cord
c. Spinal cord compression
d. Cauda equina compression
e. Anterior spinal artery occlusion

245) A 65-year-old man presents with a 2-month history of vague lower abdominal pain, diarrhoea alternating with constipation and a 4-kg weight loss. He has passed a small amount of dark-red blood per rectum. There is anaemia. The most likely diagnosis is:

a. Diverticular disease
b. Crohn's disease
c. Ulcerative colitis
d. Angiodysplasia
e. Carcinoma of the colon

246) The most useful investigation is:

a. Flexible sigmoidoscopy
b. Barium enema
c. CT scan of the abdomen
d. Abdominal ultrasonography
e. Selective mesenteric angiography

247) A 70-year-old long-sighted woman presents to A&E at midnight with vomiting that began 3 h earlier and slightly worsening vision. The eyeball is rock hard on palpation. The conjunctiva is injected. The most likely diagnosis is:

a. Acute angle-closure glaucoma
b. Anterior uveitis
c. Choroiditis
d. Retinal vein thrombosis
e. Temporal arteritis

248) A 55-year-old man who drinks heavily presents with numbness and paraesthesiae in his feet. He complains of 'walking on cotton wool'. The likely cause is:

a. Lead poisoning
b. Amyloidosis
c. Sarcoidosis
d. Vitamin B_1 deficiency
e. Vitamin B_{12} deficiency

249) A 60-year-old man presents to A&E with fever and neck pain on passively moving the chin towards the chest. Lumbar puncture shows:

White cells	3000/mL, predominantly neutrophils
Red blood cells	1/mL
Glucose	1.5 mmol/L
Protein	5 g/L

The most likely organism is:

a. *Mycobacterium tuberculosis*
b. *Neisseria meningitidis*
c. *Haemophilus influenzae*
d. *Listeria monocytogenes*
e. *Streptococcus pneumoniae*

250) A 20-year-old woman is referred for recurrent epistaxis and bruising. She takes no medication. On examination she has no facial rash or lymphadenopathy. Her spleen is mildly enlarged, and she has generalized bruising but no bone or joint tenderness. Immediate blood test results are:

White cell count	53×10^9/L
Hb	10 g/dL
Platelets	253×10^9/L
ESR	55 mm/h
MCV	90 fL
MCH	30 pg
MCHC	34 g/dL
Prolonged bleeding time	
Serum urea	6 mmol/L

The next most useful investigation would be:

a. Bone marrow aspirate
b. Haemoglobin electrophoresis
c. Platelet autoantibodies
d. Factor VIII:C and factor VIII:vWF (von Willebrand's factor) assays
e. Platelet aggregation studies

251) The most likely diagnosis is:

a. Thrombotic thrombocytopenic purpura
b. Idiopathic thrombocytopenic purpura
c. Aplastic anaemia
d. SLE
e. Von Willebrand's disease

252) A 70-year-old man presents with confusion and urinary incontinence. He is pale and his BP is 160/100. On examination the bladder is palpable to the level of the umbilicus. Rectal examination confirms an enlarged prostate. There is also peripheral oedema. Blood tests show:

White cell count	73×10^9/L
Hb	8 g/dL
Platelets	1003×10^9/L
Serum sodium	125 mmol/L
Serum potassium	6 mmol/L
Serum urea	60 mmol/L
Serum calcium	3.4 mmol/L

The diagnosis is:

a. Chronic renal failure
b. Acute renal failure
c. Benign prostatic hypertrophy
d. Prostate carcinoma
e. Myelomatosis

253) The antihypertensive drug, amlodipine, is a:

a. Calcium channel blocker
b. ACE-inhibitor
c. Potassium channel blocker
d. Loop diuretic
e. β blocker

254) A 22-year-old woman is noted to have both microcytic and macrocytic anaemia. She gives a history of intermittent diarrhoea with difficulty in flushing the stools. The most likely diagnosis is:

a. Cystic fibrosis
b. Irritable bowel syndrome
c. Coeliac disease
d. Crohn's disease
e. Ulcerative colitis

255) A 40-year-old woman on chemotherapy for metastatic breast carcinoma now presents with painful swallowing. On examination she has white plaques on top of friable mucosa in her mouth and more seen on OGD. The treatment for her dysphagia is:

a. Antispasmodics
b. Antifungal therapy
c. H_2-receptor antagonist
d. Intravenous antibiotics and analgesia
e. Dilatation of the lower oesophageal sphincter

256) A 20-year-old man presents with morning back stiffness. He has a history of iritis. On examination he has an early diastolic murmur. His chest radiograph shows bilateral diffuse reticulonodular shadowing. The most likely diagnosis is:

a. Reiter's syndrome
b. Crohn's disease
c. Rheumatoid arthritis
d. Ankylosing spondylitis
e. Sacroiliitis

257) An asymptomatic 60-year-old man is found to have an isolated raised alkaline phosphatase on routine biochemistry. Serum calcium and phosphate levels are normal. The most likely diagnosis is:

a. Osteomalacia
b. Multiple myeloma
c. Paget's disease
d. Cirrhosis
e. Hyperparathyroidism

258) The most suitable treatment for *Clostridium difficile* is:

a. Vancomycin
b. Amoxicillin
c. Gentamicin
d. Cimetidine
e. Tetracycline

259) What would be the most suitable laxative to offer a terminally ill patient hooked up to a diamorphine syringe driver?

a. Lactulose
b. Co-danthromer
c. Loperamide
d. Methylcellulose
e. Phosphate enema

260) A 50-year-old man with type 1 diabetes is started on enalapril for hypertension. Two weeks later his U&E results are noted to be abnormal. What is the most likely cause?

a. Renal papillary necrosis
b. Hypovolaemia
c. Addison's disease
d. Renal artery stenosis
e. Renal tumour

261) A dockyard worker is referred to the chest clinic for breathlessness. His chest radiograph shows pleural thickening and calcification (pleural plaques). What is the next investigation of choice?

a. Spirometry (lung function tests)
b. Arterial blood gas
c. Pulse oximetry
d. CT scan of the chest
e. PEFR (peak expiratory flow rate)

262) What is the best treatment for his condition?

a. Prednisolone
b. Salbutamol inhaler
c. Beclometasone inhaler
d. Ipratropium inhaler
e. Antituberculous chemotherapy

263) A 60-year-old man is found to have a BP of 170/100. He also has a history of asthma. What is the most appropriate drug of choice?

a. Furosemide
b. Atenolol
c. GTN spray
d. Enalapril
e. Hydralazine

264) The following medication may be offered to a man suffering from alcoholism EXCEPT:

a. Vitamin B complex
b. Thiamine
c. Diazepam
d. Heminevrin
e. Acamprosate

265) The following blood tests should routinely be offered to intravenous drug abusers EXCEPT:

a. HIV
b. Hepatitis C
c. Hepatitis B
d. LFTs
e. Hepatitis A

266) A 40-year-old man presents complaining of an episode of blacking out behind the wheel of his car. The following advice should be given to the patient EXCEPT:

a. Not to drive
b. To leave the door unlocked when bathing
c. Not to take hot baths
d. Not to iron
e. Never to be alone

267) A 60-year-old man presents with brown pigmented plaques in the axilla. He underwent prostatectomy recently. The diagnosis is likely to be:

a. Dermatitis herpetiformis
b. Pemphigoid
c. Lichen planus
d. Psoriasis
e. Acanthosis nigricans

268) A 55-year-old woman presents with severe heartburn. The pain is retrosternal and worse on stooping and after large meals. Initial investigations should include all of the following EXCEPT:

a. FBC
b. ESR
c. *Helicobacter pylori* antibody test
d. Folate and vitamin B$_{12}$ levels
e. Endoscopy

269) Initial management may include each of the following EXCEPT:

a. Quit smoking
b. Use antacids
c. Start esomeprazole
d. Start lansoprazole
e. Start triple therapy

270) You are on your way to hospital to do a night shift and find an unconscious man on the street. He is unkempt and has needle tracks on his arms and neck. He has pinpoint pupils. He is not rousable. There is no one else on the street. The most appropriate action would be:

a. Confirm that the patient is breathing, place him in the recovery position and call 999
b. Give two breaths and call 999 on your mobile to alert the paramedics that it is a probable drug overdose
c. Check that the patient is breathing and has a pulse and proceed to work
d. Run into the hospital and grab a stretcher
e. Undress the man to examine him properly for signs of trauma

271) He is transported to your A&E. The next step is:

   a. Administer naloxone i.m. only after confirmation of presence of opiates in urine
   b. Administer naloxone i.m. immediately
   c. Administer glucagon i.m.
   d. Administer intravenous fluids
   e. Arrange for urgent CT scan of the head

272) An elderly man presents with a warm swollen metatarso-phalangeal joint after a total hip replacement. The likely diagnosis is:

   a. Rheumatoid arthritis
   b. Gout
   c. Systemic sclerosis
   d. Osteoarthritis
   e. Septic arthritis

273) A 50-year-old man requests hepatitis B immunization. Pre-Hep B vaccine blood results are:

   – hepatitis B surface antigen (HBsAg)
   – hepatitis B core IgM
   – hepatitis Be antigen (HBeAg)
   + hepatitis Be antibody (HBeAb)
   + hepatitis B core antibody (total) (HBcAb)
   + hepatitis B surface antibody (HBsAb)

   How do you interpret this result?

   a. The patient has natural immunity to hepatitis B and does not require immunization
   b. The patient has had infection with hepatitis B some time in the past
   c. The patient has an acute infection with hepatitis B
   d. The patient is a chronic carrier of high infectivity
   e. The patient is a chronic carrier of low infectivity

274) The drug of choice for scabies is:

   a. Permethrin cream
   b. Malathion lotion
   c. Crotamiton
   d. Ketoconazole
   e. Mebendazole

275) Scabies is transmitted through:

   a. Bedding
   b. Towels
   c. Direct skin contact
   d. Clothing
   e. Hair

276) Causes of transient loss of consciousness include all of the following EXCEPT:

a. Reflex-mediated syncope
b. Aortic stenosis
c. Second-degree heart block
d. Subarachnoid haemorrhage
e. Hyperglycaemia

277) A 40-year-old man complains of constant, right-sided headache with severe throbbing orbital pain. The pain lasts for an hour. He also complains of watery eyes and a runny nose. He has had several episodes in the last few months and is worried that he may have a brain tumour. The most likely diagnosis is:

a. Acute sinusitis
b. Migraine headache
c. Cluster headache
d. Orbital cellulitis
e. Hayfever

278) A 65-year-old woman complains of severe right-sided headache, centred in the eye, with nausea and vomiting. On examination the conjunctiva is injected with a cloudy anterior chamber. The globe is firm and tender. The most likely diagnosis is:

a. Acute sinusitis
b. Temporal arteritis
c. Acute narrow-angle glaucoma
d. Trigeminal neuralgia
e. Periorbital abscess

279) A 50-year-old man complains of episodes of squeezing substernal chest pain when walking the dog in the morning. The attack peaks at 10 min and stops at rest. The most likely diagnosis is:

a. Oesophageal spasm
b. Costochondritis
c. Acute myocardial infarction
d. Stable angina
e. Reflux oesophagitis

280) The risk factors for coronary artery disease include all of the following EXCEPT:

a. Tobacco
b. Alcohol
c. Raised LDL-cholesterol
d. Diabetes
e. Hypertension

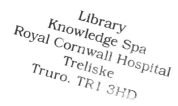

281) A 30-year-old man presents with substernal chest pain and shortness of breath. On examination he has a loud systolic ejection murmur. The Valsalva manoeuvre increases the murmur and leg raising decreases the murmur and symptoms. The most likely diagnosis is:

a. Mitral valve prolapse
b. Hypertrophic cardiomyopathy
c. Pericarditis
d. Aortic dissection
e. Stable angina

282) A 22-year-old man presents with severe, sharp chest pain that worsens with breathing. He has shallow breathing and leans toward the left side. Temperature is 39°C, BP 100/60 and pulse 120. White cell count is raised with neutrophilia. Chest radiograph is normal. The most likely diagnosis is:

a. Pulmonary embolus
b. Pleurodynia
c. Tension pneumothorax
d. Pericarditis
e. Costochondritis

283) Initial management for coma in the emergency setting may include all of the following EXCEPT:

a. 50% dextrose 50 mL i.v.
b. 2 mg naloxone i.v.
c. 100 mg thiamine i.v.
d. Assess airway, breathing and circulation (ABC)
e. Skull radiograph

284) The patient is still unresponsive. The left pupil is now dilated and unresponsive. The next step is:

a. Obtain an urgent neurosurgical consult and consider mannitol
b. Administer intravenous broad-spectrum antibiotics
c. Perform a lumbar puncture
d. Arrange an urgent EEG
e. Arrange an urgent MRI of the head

285) A 40-year-old woman presents comatose. On examination she has a left mastectomy scar. ECG shows a shortened Q–T interval. The diagnosis is:

a. Hypernatraemia
b. Hypercalcaemia
c. Addison's disease
d. Hypoglycaemia
e. Hypermagnesaemia

286) A 30-year-old woman presents with severe lethargy, weakness and abdominal pain. On examination there is hyperpigmentation of the skin folds and breast areolar areas. Blood tests reveal hypoglycaemia and hyperkalaemia. The most likely diagnosis is:

a. Conversion disorder
b. Cushing's disease
c. Addison's disease
d. Myxoedema
e. Uraemia

287) Beck's triad is:

a. Hypotension, muffled heart sounds and jugular vein distension
b. Jugular vein distension, hypertension and peripheral oedema
c. Pericardial rub, hypotension and jugular vein distension
d. Increasing blood pressure, decreasing pulse rate and shallow breathing
e. Jaundice, rigors and tender hepatomegaly

288) Lyme disease is associated with:

a. *Borrelia burgdorferi*
b. *Rickettsia rickettsii*
c. *Coxiella burnetii*
d. *Leptospira interrogans*
e. *Borrelia recurrentis*

289) Treatment for Lyme disease is:

a. Tetracycline
b. Penicillin
c. Erythromycin
d. Imipenem
e. Ciprofloxacin

290) The following conditions may be treated with chemotherapy EXCEPT:

a. Choriocarcinoma
b. Hodgkin's disease
c. Testicular carcinoma
d. Wilms' tumour
e. Adenocarcinoma of the stomach

291) Bone metastasis may occur with the following carcinomas EXCEPT:

a. Breast
b. Prostate
c. Thyroid
d. Adrenal
e. Renal

292) A 55-year-old woman presents with stridor and difficulty swallowing after a thyroidectomy. On examination, she has a tense swelling over the surgical site. Immediate course of action is:

a. Cardioversion
b. Intramuscular adrenaline
c. Needle aspiration
d. Endotracheal intubation
e. Cricothyroidotomy

293) Crohn's disease is associated with all of the following EXCEPT:

a. Rose-thorn ulcers on barium enema
b. Cobblestoning on barium enema
c. Perianal abscess
d. Loss of haustra on barium enema
e. Lymphoma

294) The most common cause of a breast mass in women under 30 is:

a. Fibrocystic disease
b. Fibroadenoma
c. Cystosarcoma phylloides
d. Breast abscess
e. Ductal carcinoma

295) Management of deep venous thrombosis include all of the following EXCEPT:

a. Check platelet count every 3 days
b. Aim for PTT (prothrombin time) at least 1.5 times normal
c. Elevate lower extremity
d. Give loading dose of 5000 U heparin followed by heparin infusion of up to 2000 U/h
e. 5000 U fragmin s.c. twice daily

296) The most common anterior mediastinal tumour in adults is:

a. Thymoma
b. Lymphoma
c. Mesothelioma
d. Myoma
e. Fibroma

297) A 55-year-old patient who smokes complains of left leg pain when walking. The pain is relieved on rest. You are unable to palpate the DP (dorsalis pedis) or PT (posterior tibial) pulses on the left. The next step is:

a. Measure ankle brachial pressures to determine ankle brachial pressure index (ABPI)
b. Arrange Doppler ultrasonography of leg
c. Arrange angiogram
d. Arrange plethysmography
e. Prescribe pentoxifylline

298) Indications for the use of octreotide (somatostatin analogue) include all of the following EXCEPT:

a. Acromegaly
b. Variceal bleeding
c. Prevention of complications after pancreatic surgery
d. Cystic fibrosis
e. Carcinoid tumour

299) On auscultation, a patient is noted to have a rumbling diastolic murmur at the apex. The murmur is accentuated during exercise. The diagnosis is:

a. Atrial fibrillation
b. Aortic regurgitation
c. Mitral regurgitation
d. Mitral stenosis
e. Pulmonary stenosis

300) A 25-year-old woman who is an intravenous drug abuser presents with an overdose on rocks (cocaine). ECG shows supraventricular tachycardia (SVT). First-line treatment for SVT is:

a. Adenosine
b. Amiodarone
c. Lidocaine
d. Procainamide
e. Verapamil

1. Medicine: EMQ Questions

Theme: investigation of tumours

Options

A. α-Fetoprotein
B. Terminal deoxyribonucleotidyltransferase (TdT)
C. Carcinoembyonic antigen (CEA)
D. Placental alkaline phosphatase (ALP)
E. Human chorionic gonadotrophin (hCG)
F. Oestrogen receptor (ER)
G. Prostate-specific antigen (PSA)
H. Basal cell carcinoma (BCC)
I. Squamous cell carcinoma (SCC) antigen
J. Calcitonin
K. Cancer antigen 125 (CA-125)

For each presentation below, choose the SINGLE most discriminating tumour marker from the list of options. Each option may be used once, more than once or not at all.

1) A 60-year-old man presents with a firm prostate nodule. He is confirmed to have prostate carcinoma on biopsy.

2) A 45-year-old man presents with a thyroid swelling. Fine-needle aspiration reveals medullary carcinoma.

3) A 60-year-old woman presents with hepatomegaly, weight loss and jaundice. Abdominal ultrasonography reveals hepatic carcinoma.

4) A 65-year-old woman presents with back pain and increasing abdominal girth. She is found to have an epithelial tumour of one ovary.

5) A 30-year-old man presents with an enlarged, smooth, firm testes. He is found to have had a seminoma following orchidectomy.

Theme: causes of dysphagia

Options

A. Achalasia
B. Pharyngeal pouch
C. Diffuse oesophageal spasm
D. Globus pharyngeus
E. Plummer–Vinson syndrome
F. Carcinoma of the oesophagus
G. Peptic stricture
H. Myasthenia gravis
I. Swallowed foreign body
J. Caustic stricture
K. Retrosternal goitre

For each presentation below, choose the SINGLE most likely cause from the list of options. Each option may be used once, more than once or not at all.

6) A 32-year-old woman presents with progressive dysphagia with regurgitation of fluids. She denies weight loss.

7) A 27-year-old man with a history of depression presents with acute dysphagia. He has a prior history of repeated suicide attempts. There are associated burns in his oropharynx.

8) A 60-year-old woman presents with progressive dysphagia. On examination she has a smooth tongue, koilonychia and iron-deficiency anaemia.

9) A 75-year-old man presents with regurgitation of food, dysphagia, halitosis and a sensation of a 'lump in the throat'.

10) A 70-year-old man presents with a short history of dysphagia and weight loss, and has palpable neck nodes on examination.

Theme: investigation of weight loss

Options

A. Stool for cysts, ova and parasites
B. Urea and electrolytes (U&Es)
C. Chest radiograph
D. Full blood count (FBC)
E. Serum glucose
F. Urinalysis
G. Thyroid function tests (TFTs)
H. Ultrasonography of abdomen
I. Barium swallow
J. Blood cultures
K. Plasma ACTH and cortisol

For each presentation below, choose the SINGLE most discriminating investigation from the list of options. Each option may be used once, more than once or not at all.

11) A 60-year-old man recently treated for renal tuberculosis presents with weight loss, diarrhoea, anorexia and hypotension, and is noted to have hyperpigmented buccal mucosa and hand creases.

12) A 50-year-old woman presents with weight loss, increased appetite, sweating, palpitations, preference for cold weather, hot, moist palms and tremors.

13) A 25-year-old man presents with steatorrhoea, diarrhoea and weight loss after eating contaminated food.

14) A 65-year-old man presents with a sudden onset of diabetes, anorexia, weight loss, and epigastric and back pain.

15) A 70-year-old woman presents with progressive dysphagia, weight loss and a sensation of food sticking in her throat.

Theme: investigation of pyrexia of unknown origin

Options

A. Haemoglobin
B. FBC
C. ESR
D. Lymph node biopsy
E. CT scan of the chest
F. Stool cultures
G. Mantoux test
H. Monospot
I. Echocardiography for vegetations
J. Kveim's test
K. HIV antibody titres

For each presentation below, choose the SINGLE most discriminating investigation from the list of options. Each option may be used once, more than once or not at all.

16) A 17-year-old boy presents with a 2-week history of fever, malaise and cervical lymphadenopathy. On examination there is tenderness in the right upper quadrant of the abdomen and the sclerae are yellow.

17) A 25-year-old man who is drug addicted presents with a low-grade fever, malaise, a change in heart murmur, splinter haemorrhages in the nailbeds and Osler's nodes in the finger pulp.

18) A 54-year-old man presents with a 2-month history of unilateral enlargement of his right tonsil, fluctuating pyrexia and multiple neck nodes.

19) A 25-year-old woman presents with fever, malaise, erythema nodosum and polyarthralgia. The chest radiograph reveals mediastinal hilar lymphadenopathy.

20) A 29-year-old man who is an intravenous drug abuser presents with fever and a neck node discharging a cheesy, malodorous substance.

Theme: treatment of meningitis

Options

A. Benzylpenicillin
B. Chloramphenicol
C. Ampicillin
D. Rifampicin, ethambutol, isoniazid and pyrazinamide
E. Amphotericin B and flucytosine
F. Gentamicin
G. Erythromycin
H. Cefotaxime
I. Oral rifampicin
J. Vancomycin
K. Supportive

For each case below, choose the SINGLE most appropriate treatment from the list of options. Each option may be used once, more than once or not at all.

21) A 3-year-old girl presents with acute onset of pyrexia, nausea and vomiting. Lumbar puncture reveals high protein and polymorph count and low glucose. Gram-negative bacilli are present in the smear and culture.

22) A 40-year-old man presents with fever and meningeal signs. Lumbar puncture reveals 20/mm^3 of mononuclear cells, 2 g/L of protein and a glucose level half the plasma level. There are no organisms in the smear.

23) A 17-year-old girl presents with fever, odd behaviour, purpura and conjunctival petechiae. Lumbar puncture reveals Gram-negative cocci.

24) A 22-year-old man presents with fever, headache and drowsiness. Lumbar puncture reveals 1000 mononuclear cells/mm^3, 0.5 g/L of protein and a glucose more than two-thirds of the plasma glucose level. Organisms are absent.

25) The 25-year-old husband of a patient admitted with pyogenic meningitis admits to having oral contact with his wife and is anxious.

Theme: causes of anaemia

Options

A. Vitamin B_{12} deficiency
B. Iron deficiency
C. Sickle cell anaemia
D. Pernicious anaemia
E. Autoimmune haemolytic anaemia
F. Hypothyroidism
G. Sideroblastic anaemia
H. Anaemia of chronic disease
I. Glucose-6-phosphate dehydrogenase deficiency
J. Thalassaemia
K. Coeliac disease

For each presentation below, choose the SINGLE most likely cause from the list of options. Each option may be used once, more than once or not at all.

26) An 8-year-old boy presents with painful swelling of the hands and feet, jaundice and anaemia. He is noted to have splenomegaly. A blood film shows target cells.

27) A 6-month-old baby boy presents with severe anaemia and failure to thrive. Blood film shows target cells, and hypochromic and microcytic cells. HbF persists.

28) A 40-year-old woman presents with fatigue, dyspnoea, paraesthesiae and a sore red tongue. Blood film shows hypersegmented polymorphs, an MCV >110 fL and a low Hb.

29) A 60-year-old man post-gastrectomy presents with macrocytic anaemia. He drinks alcohol regularly.

30) A 22-year-old Greek man presents with rapid anaemia and jaundice after treatment for malaria. He is noted to have Heinz bodies.

Theme: diagnosis of red eye

Options

A. Acute glaucoma
B. Iritis
C. Conjunctivitis
D. Subconjunctival haemorrhage
E. Optic neuritis
F. Conjunctival haemorrhages
G. Scleritis
H. Anterior uveitis
I. Posterior uveitis
J. Retinal haemorrhages

For each patient below, choose the SINGLE most likely diagnosis from the list of options. Each option may be used once, more than once or not at all.

31) A 55-year-old woman presents with an entirely red right eye. The iris is injected, and the pupil is fixed and dilated. The intraocular pressure is high.

32) A 20-year-old man presents with a non-tender red eye. On examination the sclera is bright red with a white rim around the limbus. The iris, pupil, cornea and intraocular pressure are normal.

33) A 33-year-old woman presents with a painful red eye. The conjunctival vessels are injected and blanch on pressure. The iris, pupil, cornea and intraocular pressure are normal.

34) A 40-year-old man presents with redness most marked around the cornea. The colour does not blanch on pressure. The iris is injected, and the pupil is small and fixed. The cornea and intraocular pressure are normal.

35) A 20-year-old man with non-specific urethritis and seronegative arthritis is also noted to have red eye associated with Reiter's syndrome.

Theme: diagnosis of skin manifestations of systemic diseases

Options

A. Erythema nodosum
B. Erythema multiforme
C. Erythema marginatum
D. Erythema chronicum migrans
E. Vitiligo
F. Pyoderma gangrenosum
G. Acquired ichthyosis
H. Necrobiosis lipoidica
I. Dermatitis herpetiformis
J. Acanthosis nigricans
K. Pretibial myxoedema

For each patient below, choose the SINGLE most likely skin manifestation from the list of options. Each option may be used once, more than once or not at all.

36) A 53-year-old woman presents with proptosis, heat intolerance and red oedematous swellings over the lateral malleoli, which progress to thickened oedema.

37) A 45-year-old man presents with shiny area on his shins with yellowish skin and telangiectasia. He also has areas of fat necrosis.

38) A 55-year-old woman who is advised to eat a gluten-free diet presents with itchy blisters in groups on her knees, elbows and scalp.

39) A 30-year-old man with Crohn's disease presents with a pustule on his leg with a tender red–blue necrotic edge.

40) A 15-year-old girl presents with fever and mouth ulcers. She is also noted to have target lesions with a central blister on her palms and soles.

Theme: diagnosis of eye problems

Options

A. Flame-and-blot haemorrhages
B. Proliferative retinopathy
C. Xanthelasma
D. Senile cataracts
E. Amaurosis fugax
F. Optic atrophy
G. Orbital abscess
H. Corneal arcus
I. Kayser–Fleischer rings
J. Hypertensive fundus
K. Lens opacities
L. Background retinopathy

For each patient below, choose the SINGLE most likely diagnosis from the list of options. Each option may be used once, more than once or not at all.

41) A 65-year-old man with type 1 diabetes is noted to have a white ring in his cornea surrounding his iris.

42) A 55-year-old man complains of 'a curtain passing over his eyes'. Carotid bruits are present on auscultation.

43) A 12-year-old boy, following an episode of sinusitis, complains of persistent pain behind the right eye with eyelid swelling and diminished vision.

44) A 40-year-old woman complains of pruritus, jaundice and finger clubbing. There are bright yellow plaques on both eyelids.

45) A 30-year-old man is noted to have rubeosis iridis, cotton-wool spots and cluster haemorrhages.

Theme: diagnosis of haematological diseases

Options

A. Hereditary spherocytosis
B. Myeloid metaplasia
C. Uraemia
D. Iron-deficiency anaemia
E. Sickle cell anaemia
F. Megaloblastic anaemia
G. Chronic granulocytic leukaemia
H. Infectious mononucleosis
I. Chronic lymphocytic leukaemia
J. Acute myeloid leukaemia
K. Multiple myeloma
L. Hodgkin's disease

For each blood smear below, choose the SINGLE most likely diagnosis from the list of options. Each option may be used once, more than once or not at all.

46) A 25-year-old woman presents with an enlarged, painless lymph node in the neck. She also reports fever and weight loss. Peripheral blood smear shows Reed–Sternberg cells with a bilobed, mirror-imaged nucleus.

47) A 70-year-old man presents with bone pain, anaemia and renal failure. Bone marrow reveals an abundance of malignant plasma cells.

48) A 10-year-old boy presents with swelling of the hands and feet, and anaemia. Peripheral blood smear reveals target cells and elongated crescent-shaped red blood cells.

49) A 50-year-old man with type 1 diabetes presents with a 'lemon' tinge to the skin, itching, peripheral oedema, pleural effusions and anaemia. Peripheral blood smear reveals numerous Burr cells, red blood cells with spiny projections.

50) A 65-year-old woman presents with anaemia. She has koilonychia and atrophic glossitis. A blood smear reveals microcytic, hypochromic blood cells.

Theme: diagnosis of heart conditions

Options

A. Anterolateral myocardial infarction (MI)
B. Left ventricular failure
C. Atrial fibrillation
D. Acute pulmonary embolism
E. Acute pericarditis
F. Mitral stenosis
G. Right ventricular failure
H. Hypokalaemia
I. Hypocalcaemia
J. Aortic regurgitation
K. Inferolateral MI

For each presentation below, choose the SINGLE most likely diagnosis from the list of options. Each option may be used once, more than once or not at all.

51) A 60-year-old man presents with chest pain radiating down the left arm. A 12-lead ECG reveals Q waves in II, III and AVf, with T-wave changes in V5 and V6.

52) A 50-year-old woman presents with a fast heart rate with an irregular rhythm. There are no P waves on the ECG. She states that she has lost weight recently and is 'nervous'. She also suffers from palpitations.

53) On auscultation a patient is noted to have a rumbling diastolic murmur at the apex. The murmur is accentuated during exercise.

54) A 60-year-old man on digitalis and diuretics presents with weakness and lethargy. ECG shows flat T waves and prominent U waves.

55) A 65-year-old man with chronic bronchitis presents with a raised JVP, hepatomegaly, and ankle and sacral oedema.

Theme: causes of hypertension

Options

A. Coarctation of the aorta
B. Cushing's syndrome
C. Phaeochromocytoma
D. Primary hyperaldosteronism
E. Polyarteritis nodosa
F. Polycystic kidneys
G. Acromegaly
H. Pre-eclampsia
I. Essential hypertension
J. Renal artery stenosis
K. Chronic glomerulonephritis

For each presentation below, choose the SINGLE most likely cause from the list of options. Each option may be used once, more than once or not at all.

56) A 45-year-old woman presents with hypertension and confusion. She has truncal obesity, proximal myopathy and osteoporosis. The 24-hour urinary free cortisol level is raised.

57) A 35-year-old man presents with hypertension and complains of tingling in his fingers. He has an enlarged tongue and prognathism. The glucose tolerance curve is diabetic.

58) A 45-year-old woman with disproportionately long limbs presents with hypertension. Blood pressure is different on both arms and lower in the legs.

59) A 40-year-old man post-thyroidectomy for medullary thyroid carcinoma presents with hypertension and complains of attacks of severe headache and palpitations. He is noted to have glycosuria.

60) A 50-year-old man presents with hypertension, haematuria and abdominal pain. A large kidney is palpated on examination, and the diagnosis is confirmed on ultrasonography.

Theme: causes of peripheral neuropathy

Options

A. Carcinomatous neuropathy
B. Side effect of drug therapy
C. Diabetic neuropathy
D. Vitamin B_{12} deficiency
E. Vitamin B_1 deficiency
F. Polyarteritis nodosa
G. Guillain–Barré syndrome
H. Amyloidosis
I. Sarcoidosis
J. Industrial poisoning
K. Porphyria

For each patient below, choose the SINGLE most likely diagnosis from the list of options. Each option may be used once, more than once or not at all.

61) A 50-year-old man presents with distal sensory neuropathy affecting the lower limbs in a 'stocking' distribution and is noted to have Charcot's joints. The ankle reflex is absent.

62) A 55-year-old man who drinks heavily presents with numbness and paraesthesiae in his feet. He complains of 'walking on cotton wool'.

63) A 40-year-old man, who is being treated with chemotherapy for lymphoma, presents with peripheral paraesthesiae, loss of deep tendon reflexes and abdominal bloating.

64) A 45-year-old woman presents with peripheral neuropathy. There is bilateral hilar gland enlargement on the chest radiograph. The Mantoux test is negative. She also suffers from polyarthralgia and has tender, red, raised lesions on her shin.

65) A 25-year-old man presents with paraesthesiae followed by a flaccid paralysis of his limbs and face. He has a history of a recent upper respiratory tract infection.

Theme: diagnosis of pulmonary diseases

Options

A. Pneumoconiosis
B. Cystic fibrosis
C. Mycoplasma pneumonia
D. Adult respiratory distress syndrome
E. Pulmonary contusion
F. Carcinoma of the bronchus
G. Pancoast's tumour
H. Bilateral bronchopneumonia
I. Sarcoidosis
J. Tuberculosis

For each case below, choose the SINGLE most likely diagnosis from the list of options. Each option may be used once, more than once or not at all.

66) A 30-year-old woman presents with fever, pharyngitis and a cough. A chest radiograph shows widespread bilateral patchy consolidation. Cold agglutinins are detected.

67) A 40 year old with alcohol problems presents with repeated small haemoptysis and a cough with mucoid sputum. A chest radiograph shows right upper lobe consolidation and a large central cavity. The Heaf test is positive.

68) A 60-year-old man presents with dyspnoea and a cough. A radiograph shows extensive pulmonary fibrosis, bilateral pleural thickening and pleural calcification.

69) A 14-year-old boy presents with repeated lower tract respiratory infections. On examination there is finger clubbing. He has weight loss and steatorrhoea. The radiograph shows bronchial wall thickening, ring shadows of bronchiectasis and widespread ill-defined shadowing.

70) A 40-year-old man presents with cough and haemoptysis. The radiograph shows a right hilar mass and a patch of consolidation in the right upper lobe laterally.

Theme: treatment of hypertension

Options

A. Atenolol
B. Bendrofluazide
C. Furosemide
D. Methyldopa
E. Amlodipine
F. Nifedipine
G. Hydralazine
H. Captopril
I. Sodium nitroprusside
J. Lisinopril
K. Non-drug treatment

For each patient below, choose the SINGLE most appropriate treatment from the list of options. Each option may be used once, more than once or not at all.

71) A 60-year-old man presents with a BP of 165/95. He is asymptomatic and all investigations are normal.

72) A 55-year-old man with type 1 diabetes presents to his GP with a BP of 170/110. The blood pressure is consistently high on subsequent visits despite conservative measures. Blood tests are normal.

73) A 50-year-old man with asthma presents to his GP with a BP of 180/120. All underlying causes have been excluded.

74) A 60-year-old man is brought into A&E complaining of severe headaches. On arrival he has a seizure. His BP is noted to be 220/140 and, on fundoscopic examination, there is papilloedema.

75) A 66-year-old man on atenolol 100 mg once daily continues to have a diastolic BP of 115. He also takes allopurinol. A second drug is recommended.

Theme: causes of splenomegaly

Options

A. Typhoid
B. Gaucher's disease
C. Malaria
D. Schistosomiasis
E. Lymphoma
F. Leishmaniasis
G. Idiopathic thrombocytopenic purpura
H. Polycythaemia rubra vera
I. Felty's syndrome
J. Leptospirosis
K. Chronic myeloid leukaemia

For each case below, choose the SINGLE most likely cause from the list of options. Each option may be used once, more than once or not at all.

76) A 20-year-old man presents acutely with fever, jaundice, purpura, injected conjunctiva and painful calves after swimming outdoors.

77) A 26-year-old man recently returned from a trip to India presents with intermittent fevers, cough, diarrhoea, epistaxis and massive splenomegaly.

78) A 22-year-old woman presents with epistaxis and easy bruising. On examination the spleen is palpable.

79) A 30-year-old Jewish man presents with incidental splenomegaly on a routine physical examination at his GP's clinic. Serum acid phosphatase is elevated. He admits to having episodes of bone pain. His uncle also has an enlarged spleen.

80) A 60-year-old woman with rheumatoid arthritis presents with splenomegaly. Full blood count shows a white cell count of 1500/mm^3.

Theme: causes of haematuria

Options

A. Ureteric calculus
B. Acute pyelonephritis
C. Benign prostatic hypertrophy
D. Acute cystitis
E. Malaria
F. Carcinoma of the kidney
G. Bladder carcinoma
H. Bilharzia
I. Prostate carcinoma
J. Renal vein thrombosis
K. Acute intermittent porphyria

For each of the cases below, choose the SINGLE most likely cause from the list of options. Each option may be used once, more than once or not at all.

81) An 18-year-old young woman started on oral contraceptives complains of colicky abdominal pain and vomiting and fever. Urine is positive for red blood cells and protein. She develops progressive weakness in her extremities.

82) A 60-year-old man presents with intermittent colicky loin pain and night sweats. He has profuse haematuria with passage of blood clots. He is noted to have a varicocele and peripheral oedema. He admits to loss of energy and weight loss.

83) A 25-year-old woman presents with fever and tachycardia. On examination the renal angle is very tender. Urine is cloudy and blood stained.

84) A 40-year-old man complains of severe colicky loin pain that radiates to his scrotum. He is noted to have microscopic haematuria. No masses are palpated.

85) A 60-year-old man complains of increased frequency of micturition with suprapubic ache. Urine is cloudy and mahogany brown in colour.

Theme: causes of abnormal ECGs

Options

A. Hypokalaemia
B. Hyperkalaemia
C. Hypocalcaemia
D. Hypercalcaemia
E. Myocardial ischaemia
F. Inferior MI
G. Acute pulmonary embolism
H. Acute pericarditis
I. Atrial fibrillation
J. Myxoedema
K. Digitalis intoxication
L. Inferolateral MI

For each case below, choose the SINGLE most likely cause of ECG changes from the list of options. Each option may be used once, more than once or not at all.

86) A 60-year-old woman taking furosemide is noted to have 'U' waves in leads V3 and V4.

87) A 50-year-old man presents with fever and chest pain. He has a history of angina. ECG reveals concave elevation of the ST segments in leads II, V5 and V6.

88) A 55-year-old man presents with chest pain and dyspnoea. ECG reveals 'Q' waves in leads III and AVf, and inverted 'T' waves in leads V1−3.

89) A 55-year-old woman who has undergone thyroidectomy is noted to have an ECG with a Q−T interval of 0.50.

90) A 60-year-old woman presents with hoarseness. She is a smoker and is on Prozac. Pulse rate is 44/min and ECG is noted for sinus bradycardia and reduced amplitude of P, QRS and T waves in all leads.

Theme: treatment of medical emergencies

Options

A. Cardioversion
B. Cricothyroidotomy
C. Needle thoracocentesis
D. Needle pericardiocentesis
E. Insertion of chest drain
F. Endotracheal intubation
G. Defibrillation
H. Needle aspiration
I. Intravenous heparin
J. Intramuscular adrenaline
K. Intravenous aminophylline

For each case below, choose the SINGLE most appropriate treatment from the list of options. Each option may be used once, more than once or not at all.

91) A 45-year-old woman presents with acute dyspnoea and stridor. The tongue is swollen.

92) A 20-year-old student presents with respiratory distress and pleuritic pain. On examination there are distended neck veins and no breath sounds over the right lung field.

93) A 30-year-old man presents with chest pain. There are distended neck veins and muffled heart sounds. Blood pressure is 80/50.

94) A 55-year-old woman presents with stridor and difficulty swallowing following a thyroidectomy. On examination there is a tense swelling over the surgical site.

95) A 30-year-old woman presents with acute dyspnoea and pleuritic pain. Regular medications include salbutamol inhaler and Microgynon. Respiratory rate is 30 with a small-volume, rapid pulse rate of 110 and a BP of 80/50. The JVP is raised. Chest radiograph is normal. ECG shows sinus tachycardia.

Theme: investigation of liver disease

Options

A. Mitochondrial antibodies
B. Serum iron and total iron-binding capacity
C. Serum copper and ceruloplasmin
D. Serum bilirubin and liver function tests
E. HBsAg
F. Hepatitis C IgG
G. Antibodies against nuclei and actin
H. Antibodies to HAV
I. γ-Glutamyltransferase level
J. α₁-Antitrypsin

For each presentation below, choose the SINGLE most discriminating investigation from the list of options. Each option may be used once, more than once or not at all.

96) A 60-year-old man with emphysema presents with liver disease. The sputum is purulent and found to contain elastases and proteases.

97) A 50-year-old woman presents with pruritus and jaundice. She complains of dry eyes and mouth. Xanthelasma and hepatosplenomegaly are present on examination.

98) A 50-year-old well-bronzed man presents with a loss of libido. On examination hepatomegaly is noted. He takes Humulin and Actrapid insulin.

99) A 22-year-old man presents with tremor and dysarthria. On examination he is noted to have a greenish-brown pigment at the corneoscleral junction.

100) A 30-year-old woman presents with acute hepatitis. She is pyrexial, jaundiced, with hepatosplenomegaly, bruising and migratory polyarthritis. She is noted to have a goitre.

Theme: causes of back pain

Options

A. Multiple myeloma
B. Secondary prostate disease
C. Osteomyelitis
D. Ankylosing spondylitis
E. Sarcoidosis
F. Lupus
G. Reiter's disease
H. Lumbar prolapse and sciatica
I. Spondylolisthesis
J. Spinal stenosis
K. Paget's disease
L. Osteoarthritis

For each presentation below, choose the SINGLE most likely cause from the list of options. Each option may be used once, more than once or not at all.

101) A 30-year-old woman complains of sudden and severe back pain. Her back has 'gone'. She walks with a compensated scoliosis. On examination she has pain from the buttock to her ankle and sensory loss over the sole of her left foot and calf.

102) A 50-year-old man presents with back pain radiating down the back of both his legs. The pain is aggravated by walking and relieved by resting or leaning forward. On examination he has limited straight-leg raise and absent ankle reflexes.

103) A 50-year-old woman presents with backache. She is noted to have a normocytic, normochromic anaemia and a high ESR.

104) A 60-year-old man presents with lumbar spine bone pain and pain in his hips. The serum alkaline phosphatase is 1000 IU/L. The calcium and phosphate levels are normal. He is hard of hearing.

105) A 20-year-old man complains of lower back pain radiating down the back of both his legs. On a radiograph the vertebrae are square and tramline. ESR is elevated.

Theme: investigation of urinary tract obstruction

Options

A. Excretion urography
B. Ultrasonography
C. Dynamic scintigraphy
D. Cystourethroscopy
E. Plain KUB film
F. Pressure–flow studies
G. Retrograde ureterography
H. Urethrography
I. Serum urea and electrolytes
J. Urinalysis
K. Midstream specimen for culture

For each presentation below, choose the SINGLE most discriminating investigation from the list of options. Each option may be used once, more than once or not at all.

106) A 65-year-old man with diabetes presents with a painless distended bladder. On digital rectal examination, his prostate is not enlarged.

107) A 40-year-old man presents with severe colicky loin pain radiating to his testicle. Plain abdominal radiograph is unremarkable. He has microscopic haematuria.

108) A 50-year-old man presents with severe oliguria post-kidney transplantation.

109) A 60-year-old man post-thyroidectomy presents with painful urinary retention. There is some difficulty in catheterization with a 900 mL residual. Digital rectal examination reveals a smooth, enlarged prostate.

110) A 60-year-old man presents with malaise, back pain, normochromic anaemia, uraemia and a high ESR. He is known to have carcinoma of the colon.

Theme: diagnosis of chronic joint pain

Options

A. Gout
B. Septic arthritis
C. Rheumatoid arthritis
D. Osteoarthritis
E. Pyrophosphate arthropathy
F. Systemic lupus erythematosus
G. Systemic sclerosis
H. Polymyositis
I. Still's disease
J. Multiple myeloma
K. Sjögren's syndrome

For each case below, choose the SINGLE most likely diagnosis from the list of options. Each option may be used once, more than once or not at all.

111) A 70-year-old woman complains of arthritis in the fingers and big toe. On examination there are bony swellings of the first carpometacarpal joints. The proximal interphalangeal joints and metatarsophalangeal joint are also affected.

112) A 45-year-old woman presents with swelling and stiffness of her fingers. On examination she has sausage-like fingers with flexion deformities. She is noted to have a beaked nose. She takes Losec. A radiograph of her hands reveals deposits of calcium around the fingers and erosion of the tufts of the distal phalanges.

113) A 40-year-old woman complains of arthritic hands, weakness in her arms and difficulty swallowing. She has trouble carrying her shopping. On examination the small joints of her hands are swollen. Blood tests reveal a raised ESR and a normocytic anaemia. Serum antinuclear antibodies and rheumatoid factor tests are positive.

114) A 50-year-old woman on thyroxine for hypothyroidism presents with stiff swollen knees. Aspiration of the synovial fluid reveals positively birefringent crystals.

115) An elderly man presents with a red, warm, swollen, metatarsophalangeal joint following a right total hip replacement operation.

Theme: causes of finger clubbing

Options

A. Bronchial carcinoma
B. Bronchiectasis
C. Lung abscess
D. Empyema
E. Cryptogenic fibrosing alveolitis
F. Mesothelioma
G. Cyanotic heart disease
H. Subacute bacterial endocarditis
I. Cirrhosis
J. Inflammatory bowel disease
K. Coeliac disease
L. Gastrointestinal lymphoma

For each presentation below, choose the SINGLE most likely associative cause from the list of options. Each option may be used once, more than once or not at all.

116) A 35-year-old man who is addicted to heroin presents with fever, night sweats and haematuria. On examination he is noted to have a heart murmur and finger clubbing.

117) A 50-year-old farmer is noted to have a dry cough, exertional dyspnoea, weight loss, arthralgia and finger clubbing. On the radiograph there is bilateral diffuse reticulonodular shadowing at the bases.

118) A 60-year-old man presents with severe chest pain, dyspnoea and finger clubbing. He admits to asbestos exposure 20 years ago. He denies smoking. A chest radiograph reveals a unilateral pleural effusion.

119) A 30-year-old woman presents with fever, diarrhoea and crampy abdominal pain. She is noted to have finger clubbing, anal fissures and a skin tag.

120) A 50-year-old man presents with haematemesis. He is noted to have finger clubbing, gynaecomastia and spider naevi.

Theme: causes of headache

Options

A. Meningitis
B. Migraine headache
C. Cluster headache
D. Tension headache
E. Subarachnoid haemorrhage
F. Sinusitis
G. Benign intracranial hypertension
H. Cervical spondylosis
I. Giant-cell arteritis
J. Otitis media
K. Transient ischaemic attack

For each case below, choose the SINGLE most likely cause from the list of options. Each option may be used once, more than once or not at all.

121) A 25-year-old woman presents with episodes of unilateral throbbing headache, nausea and vomiting. She states that it is aggravated by light. The episodes seem to occur before menstruation.

122) A 40-year-old man presents with severe pain around his right eye with eyelid swelling lasting 20 min. He has had several attacks during the past weeks. The attacks are worse at night.

123) A 10-year-old boy presents with fever, headache, left eye pain and swelling. He described his vision as blurry. He has recently recovered from a cold.

124) A 60-year-old woman presents with bitemporal headache, unilateral blurry vision and pain on combing her hair. The ESR is elevated.

125) A 30-year-old obese woman presents with headache and diplopia. On examination she has papilloedema. She is alert with no focal symptoms and signs.

Theme: diagnosis of cardiovascular disease

Options

A. Aortic regurgitation
B. Mitral stenosis
C. Mitral regurgitation
D. Aortic stenosis
E. Atrial myxoma
F. Tricuspid regurgitation
G. Pulmonary stenosis
H. Atrial septal defect
I. Ventricular septal defect
J. Fallot's tetralogy
K. Patent ductus arteriosus
L. Coarctation of the aorta
M. Eisenmenger's syndrome

For each patient below, choose the SINGLE most likely diagnosis from the list of options. Each option may be used once, more than once or not at all.

126) A 35-year-old pregnant woman presents to her GP for her first prenatal check-up. He notes that her blood pressure differs in both arms and is lower in the legs.

127) A 13-year-old boy presents with dyspnoea and short stature. He is noted to have finger clubbing. The chest radiograph reveals a boot-shaped heart and a large aorta.

128) A preterm baby presents with tachypnoea and expiratory grunting. The baby is noted to have a continuous machinery-like murmur in the second left intercostal space and posteriorly. The ECG is normal.

129) A 33-year-old woman with Marfan's syndrome is noted to have a fixed wide split of the second heart sound. The ECG shows a partial right bundle-branch block with right axis deviation and right ventricular hypertrophy.

130) A 40-year-old person who is a drug addict is noted to have a pansystolic murmur at the bottom of the sternum. Giant 'cv' waves are present in the jugular venous pulse.

Theme: causes of pneumonia

Options

A. *Chlamydia psittaci*
B. *Streptococcus pneumoniae*
C. *Mycoplasma pneumoniae*
D. *Haemophilus influenzae*
E. *Staphylococcus aureus*
F. *Legionella pneumophila*
G. *Coxiella burnetii*
H. *Pseudomonas aeruginosa*
I. *Pneumocystis jiroveci*
J. *Aspergillus fumigatus*
K. Cytomegalovirus
L. *Actinomyces israelii*
M. *Klebsiella pneumoniae*

For each case below, choose the SINGLE most likely cause from the list of options. Each option may be used once, more than once or not at all.

131) A pet-shop owner presents with high swinging fever, cough and malaise. He has scanty rose spots over his abdomen. The chest radiograph reveals diffuse pneumonia.

132) A 70-year-old man with alcohol problems presents with sudden onset of purulent productive cough. The chest radiograph shows consolidation of the left upper lobe.

133) A 10-year-old boy with cystic fibrosis presents with pneumonia.

134) A 30-year-old man with AIDS presents with fever, dry cough and dyspnoea. The radiograph shows diffuse bilateral alveolar and interstitial shadowing starting in the perihilar regions and spreading outward.

135) A 20-year-old man who is an intravenous drug abuser presents with breathlessness and cough. The radiograph reveals patchy areas of consolidation with abscess formation.

Theme: causes of visual disturbance

Options

A. *Chlamydia trachomatis*
B. Side effect of medication
C. Giant-cell arteritis
D. Diabetic retinopathy
E. Multiple sclerosis
F. Vitamin B_{12} deficiency
G. Horner's syndrome
H. Neurosyphilis
I. Myasthenia gravis
J. Pituitary neoplasm
K. Oculomotor nerve lesion
L. Abducens nerve lesion

For each case below, choose the SINGLE most likely cause from the list of options. Each option may be used once, more than once or not at all.

136) A 40-year-old woman presents with blurry vision. On examination, when asked to look to her left, the left eye develops nystagmus and the right eye fails to adduct. When asked to look to her right, the left eye fails to adduct.

137) A 30-year-old woman is noted to have a small, irregular pupil that is fixed to light but constricts on convergence. Fasting blood glucose is 5 mmol/L.

138) A 24-year-old man presents with unilateral pupillary constriction with slight ptosis and enophthalmos. He is noted to have a cervical rib on a radiograph.

139) A 25-year-old man who has sustained head injury in an RTA presents with diplopia on lateral gaze. On examination he has a convergent squint with diplopia when looking to the left side.

140) A 40-year-old man with diabetes presents with a unilateral complete ptosis. The eye is noted to be facing down and out. The pupil is spared.

Theme: investigation of dementia

Options

A. Chest radiograph
B. Serum calcium level
C. TSH levels and serum T_4
D. Full blood count and film
E. EEG
F. Lumbar puncture
G. Serum urea
H. Liver function tests
I. CT scan
J. Serum glucose
K. VDRL
L. HIV serology
M. Serum copper and ceruloplasmin
N. Dietary history
O. Drug levels

For each case below, choose the SINGLE most discriminating investigation from the list of options. Each option may be used once, more than once or not at all.

141) A 50-year-old woman who underwent thyroidectomy a week before now presents with dementia. She also complains of perioral tingling.

142) A 70-year-old man presents with progressive dementia and tremor. On examination he has extensor plantar reflexes and Argyll Robertson pupils.

143) A 40-year-old man with a history of epilepsy presents with progressive dementia with fluctuating levels of consciousness. On examination he has unequal pupils.

144) A 30-year-old homosexual man presents with weight loss, chronic diarrhoea and progressive dementia. On examination he has purple papules on his legs.

145) A 30-year-old man presents with sweating, agitation, tremors and dementia. He admits to binge drinking.

Theme: causes of vertigo

Options

A. Migraine
B. Vestibular neuronitis
C. Multiple sclerosis
D. Lateral medullary syndrome
E. Wernicke's encephalopathy
F. Vertebrobasilar ischaemia
G. Epilepsy
H. Hypoglycaemia
I. Arrhythmias
J. Ménière's disease
K. Acoustic neuroma
L. Postural hypotension

For each case below, choose the SINGLE most likely cause from the list of options. Each option may be used once, more than once or not at all.

146) A 40-year-old man presents with vertigo, nausea, and weakness. He also complains of a tingling sensation down his right arm and double vision in one eye. On examination he has loss of central vision, nystagmus and ataxia.

147) A 50-year-old man presents with severe vertigo with vomiting and left-sided facial pain. On examination he has nystagmus on looking to the left. His soft palate is paralysed on the left side and he has analgesia to pinprick on the left side of the face and right limbs. He also has a left-sided Horner's syndrome.

148) A 50-year-old woman presents with vertigo and unilateral deafness. The attacks of vertigo last for hours and are accompanied by vomiting. On examination she has nystagmus and a low-frequency sensorineural hearing loss.

149) A 20-year-old man presents with sudden onset of vertigo and vomiting. He denies tinnitus or hearing loss. He had an upper respiratory tract infection a week ago.

150) A 60-year-old man presents with vertigo brought on by turning his head, ataxia, dysarthria and nystagmus.

Theme: treatment of respiratory diseases

Options

A. β₂-Adrenoreceptor agonist
B. Intravenous aminophylline
C. Erythromycin
D. Tobramycin and carbenicillin
E. Ciprofloxacin
F. Co-trimoxazole
G. Rifampicin and isoniazid
H. Prednisolone
I. Cyclophosphamide
J. Plasmapheresis
K. Tetracycline

For each presentation below, choose the SINGLE most appropriate treatment from the list of options. Each option may be used once, more than once or not at all.

151) A 12-year-old boy with cystic fibrosis presents with a chest infection. The boy also has mild renal failure.

152) A 40 year old who is an inpatient on a psychiatric ward presents with dry cough and confusion. Blood tests reveal lymphopenia and hyponatraemia. A chest radiograph shows right-sided lobar shadowing.

153) A 10-year-old boy presents with wheezing attacks and episodic shortness of breath. Peak expiratory flow rate is 400 L/min.

154) A 40-year-old man presents with rhinorrhoea, cough, haemoptysis and pleuritic pain. A chest radiograph shows multiple nodules.

155) A 60-year-old farmer presents with fever, cough and shortness of breath. He had been forking hay that morning. A chest radiograph shows fluffy nodular shadows in the upper zones.

Theme: investigation of haemoptysis

Options

A. FBC
B. Clotting studies
C. Bronchography
D. Chest radiograph
E. A 12-lead ECG
F. Antinuclear antibodies and free DNA
G. Anti-glomerular basement antibody in the serum
H. CT scan of the chest
I. Heaf test
J. Urinalysis
K. Pulmonary angiogram
L. Tissue biopsy
M. Sputum cytology

For each case below, choose the SINGLE most discriminating investigation from the list of options. Each option may be used once, more than once or not at all.

156) A 40-year-old man presents with recurrent epistaxis, haemoptysis and haematuria. On examination he has a nasal septal perforation and nodules on the chest radiograph.

157) A 30-year-old man presents with haemoptysis, dyspnoea and haematuria. The chest radiograph reveals bilateral alveolar infiltrates. Urinalysis shows protein and red cell casts.

158) A 60-year-old man presents with a chronic cough and mild haemoptysis. On examination he has digital clubbing with pain and swelling around his wrists. The chest radiograph reveals a single nodule.

159) A 30 year old who is an intravenous drug abuser presents with dyspnoea and haemoptysis. The chest radiograph is unremarkable and the ECG shows a sinus tachycardia with a mean P-axis shift to the right. Blood gas shows a low P_{CO_2} and an elevated pH.

160) A 50-year-old man presents with occasional haemoptysis and chronic productive cough. He has a history of recurrent pneumonia. The chest radiograph reveals peribronchial fibrosis.

Theme: causes of proteinuria

Options

A. Alport's syndrome
B. Minimal change disease
C. Lupus nephritis
D. Focal glomerulosclerosis
E. Membranoproliferative glomerulonephritis
F. Mesangial proliferative glomerulonephritis
G. Membranous glomerulonephritis
H. Idiopathic crescenteric glomerulonephritis
I. Diabetic nephropathy
J. Henoch–Schönlein purpura
K. Goodpasture's syndrome
L. Postinfectious glomerulonephritis

For each case below, choose the SINGLE most likely cause from the list of options. Each option may be used once, more than once or not at all.

161) A 40-year-old man presents with proteinuria, haematuria and progressive renal failure. He is noted to have a high-frequency sensorineural hearing loss. He has a sister who was noted to have microscopic haematuria but is asymptomatic.

162) A 7-year-old boy presents with generalized oedema and proteinuria. Electron microscopy reveals fusion of the epithelial foot processes and normal-appearing capillary and basement membranes.

163) A 30 year old who is a heroin addict presents with hypertension, oedema and oliguria, and is noted to have heavy proteinuria. A renal biopsy specimen reveals loss of glomerular cellularity and collapse of capillary loops. Adhesions between portions of the glomerular tuft and Bowman's capsule are also seen.

164) A 12-year-old boy presents with sudden onset of haematuria and oedema. Further investigations reveal proteinuria and hypocomplementaemia (C3). Subepithelial humps and foot process fusion are seen by electron microscopy.

165) A 4-year-old boy presents with a faint leg rash, bloody diarrhoea and oliguria. Further investigations reveal heavy proteinuria and an elevated serum IgA.

Theme: investigation of rheumatic diseases

Options

A. HLA B27 antigen
B. Bone scan
C. Antibody to dsDNA
D. Anti-nucleolus antibody
E. Rheumatoid factor
F. HLA DR4 antigen
G. Synovial fluid analysis with polarized light microscopy
H. Radiograph
I. Anti-centromere antibody
J. Anti-Jo-1 antibody
K. Serum uric acid
L. Anti-Ro antibody

For each case below, choose the SINGLE most discriminating investigation from the list of options. Each option may be used once, more than once or not at all.

166) A 60-year-old man with alcohol dependence presents with a hot, swollen, first metatarsophalangeal joint and a lesion on the rim of his left pinna.

167) A 65-year-old woman with a history of hypothyroidism presents with a warm, painful swollen knee with effusion. Serum calcium is normal. The radiograph reveals chondrocalcinosis.

168) A 40-year-old woman presents with flexion deformities of her fingers. She has soft-tissue swelling of her digits. She also complains of difficulty swallowing and is noted to have a beaked nose and facial telangiectasia.

169) A 30-year-old woman presents with painful digits worse in the cold and difficulty swallowing. She is noted to have tapered fingers and a fixed facial expression with facial telangiectasia. The radiograph reveals calcium around her fingers.

170) A 20-year-old woman presents with dry eyes, arthralgia, dysphagia and Raynaud's phenomenon.

Theme: causes of diarrhoea

Options

A. Campylobacter infection
B. Viral gastroenteritis
C. Ulcerative colitis
D. Crohn's disease
E. Laxative abuse
F. Pseudomembranous colitis
G. Shigella infection
H. Cryptosporidiosis infection
I. Salmonellosis
J. Irritable bowel syndrome
K. *Clostridium perfringens* infection
L. *Escherichia coli* infection

For each presentation below, choose the SINGLE most likely cause from the list of options. Each option may be used once, more than once or not at all.

171) A 30-year-old man with AIDS presents with profuse watery diarrhoea. Oocysts are detected in the stool.

172) A 25-year-old man presents with fever, bloody diarrhoea and cramping for several weeks that does not resolve with antibiotic therapy. Proctosigmoidoscopy reveals red, raw mucosa and pseudopolyps.

173) A 60-year-old man presents with fever, watery diarrhoea and crampy abdominal pain. He had completed antibiotic therapy for osteomyelitis a month ago. Proctosigmoidoscopy reveals yellowish-white plaques on the mucosa.

174) A 20-year-old man, recently back from a holiday in the Far East, presents with an abrupt onset of severe diarrhoea. The diarrhoea is self-limiting and lasts only 3 days.

175) A 20-year-old woman presents with chronic watery diarrhoea. She is emaciated. Stool electrolyte studies show an osmotic gap. Blood tests reveal hypokalaemia.

Theme: treatment of medical emergencies

Options

A. Intramuscular adrenaline
B. Emergency tracheostomy
C. Urgent endotracheal intubation
D. Type and crossmatch blood
E. Transfuse O-negative blood and apply external fixator
F. Transfer to burns unit
G. Tetanus prophylaxis
H. Intravenous antibiotics
I. Intravenous dexamethasone
J. Oxygen and nebulized salbutamol
K. Take patient straight to theatre

For each case below, choose the SINGLE most appropriate treatment from the list of options. Each option may be used once, more than once or not at all.

176) A 40-year-old pedestrian, struck by a speeding car, is brought into A&E wearing a pneumatic antishock garment for an extensive open avulsion injury to her pelvis. She is intubated with fluids running via two large-bore intravenous cannulae. She fails to respond and the blood pressure is now 65/40. The pelvis is grossly distorted.

177) A 10-year-old boy who is a burns victim is brought into A&E with worsening stridor. A facemask with 100% oxygen is covering his face, but his oxygen saturation continues to fall. His midface and mouth have been severely burned.

178) A 4-year-old girl presents with fever, stridor and dyspnoea. She is sitting forward, drooling saliva. She has no history of asthma. She is becoming more distressed.

179) An 18-year-old man presents with fever, trismus and stridor. His breathing becomes laboured with the use of accessory muscles. He becomes cyanotic. He initially presented to his GP with a sore throat a few days ago.

180) A 13 year old who is known have asthma presents with severe wheezing and a respiratory rate of 30. Pulse rate is 120.

Theme: causes of poisoning

Options

A. Lead
B. Paracetamol
C. Salicylate
D. Arsenic
E. Ethanol
F. Mercury
G. Cyanide
H. Carbon monoxide
I. Organophosphate insecticides
J. Paraquat
K. Ethylene glycol
L. Methanol

For each case below, choose the SINGLE most likely cause from the list of options. Each option may be used once, more than once or not at all.

181) A 4-year-old child presents with anorexia, nausea and vomiting. On examination he has a blue line on the gums and is noted to have a foot drop. A blood test reveals anaemia.

182) A 16-year-old girl presents with weakness, excessive salivation, vomiting, abdominal pain and diarrhoea. There is 'raindrop' pigmentation of the skin. Diagnosis is made from nail clippings.

183) A 40-year-old farmer presents with acute shortness of breath and headache. His skin is red in colour, and he smells of bitter almonds.

184) A 40-year-old woman complains of headache and memory impairment after the installation of a gas fireplace. Her skin colour is pink.

185) A 50-year-old farmer presents with nausea, vomiting, hypersalivation and bronchospasm.

Theme: treatment of diabetic complications

Options

A. Insulin sliding scale, heparin and 0.9% saline
B. Insulin sliding scale, heparin and 0.45% saline
C. Insulin sliding scale, 0.9% saline and potassium replacement
D. Insulin sliding scale, 0.45% saline and potassium replacement
E. 50 ml 50% dextrose i.v.
F. Sugary drink
G. Chest radiograph
H. Measure C-peptide levels

For each case below, choose the SINGLE most appropriate treatment from the list of options. Each option may be used once, more than once or not at all.

186) A 67-year-old man is noted to have a glucose of 37 mmol/L and a Na^+ of 163 mmol/L. He has no prior history of diabetes and has been on intravenous fluids for a week. His other medications include intravenous cefuroxime, metronidazole and dexamethasone.

187) A 60-year-old man is brought into A&E in an unconscious state. Serum glucose is 35 mmol/L. Arterial blood gas shows pH 7.2 and a $Paco_2$ 2 kPa. Serum Na^+ 140, K^+ 3.0, Cl^- 100 and HCO_3^- 5 mmol/L.

188) A 40-year-old actor with a history of diabetes is started on propranolol for stage fright. He collapses after a day shooting. He has not changed his insulin regimen. Serum glucose is 1.5 mmol/L.

189) A 50-year-old man with a history of diabetes presents in a coma. He is febrile with diminished breath sounds on auscultation. He has warm extremities. Serum glucose is 20 mmol. The white count is 22 with increased neutrophils.

190) A 50-year-old woman presents with tachycardia, sweating and agitation. Her husband has diabetes. She has a history of Munchausen's syndrome.

Theme: diagnosis of cardiovascular diseases

Options

A. Angina pectoralis
B. Aortic stenosis
C. Tricuspid regurgitation
D. Aortic regurgitation
E. Myocardial infarction
F. Acute pericarditis
G. Hypertrophic obstructive cardiomyopathy
H. Mitral regurgitation
I. Congestive cardiomyopathy
J. Mitral stenosis
K. Restrictive cardiomyopathy
L. Constrictive pericarditis
M. Dressler's syndrome

For each case below, choose the SINGLE most likely diagnosis from the list of options. Each option may be used once, more than once or not at all.

191) A 40-year-old man presents with inspiratory chest pain 2 months after a heart attack. On examination a friction rub is heard in both systole and diastole. ECG shows ST elevation throughout.

192) A 35 year old who is an intravenous drug abuser presents with right upper quadrant abdominal pain. On examination there is peripheral oedema, ascites and a pulsatile liver. On auscultation there is a holosystolic murmur along the left sternal border.

193) A 30-year-old man presents with chest pain and feeling faint. On examination there is a pansystolic murmur and a fourth heart sound. ECG shows left ventricular hypertrophy. Echocardiography shows septal hypertrophy and abnormal mitral valve motion.

194) A 40-year-old woman with Marfan's syndrome presents with shortness of breath, fainting spells and pounding of the heart. On examination there is capillary pulsation in the nailbed and pistol-shot femoral pulses. On auscultation there is a high-pitched diastolic murmur heard best at the lower left sternal edge.

195) A 40-year-old man presents after fainting during a work-out in the gym. On auscultation there is a harsh, midsystolic, cresecendo–decrescendo, systolic murmur in the aortic area radiating to the carotids.

Theme: treatment of cardiac arrhythmias

Options

A. Atropine 1 mg intravenous push
B. Precordial thump
C. CPR until a defibrillator is present
D. CPR, adrenaline 1:1000 intravenous push
E. Transvenous pacemaker
F. Defibrillate at 200 J
G. External pacemaker
H. Oxygen 4 L/min
I. Lidocaine i.v.
J. Morphine i.m.

For each patient below, choose the SINGLE most appropriate treatment from the list of options. Each option may be used once, more than once or not at all.

196) A 60-year-old man presents with chest pain and shortness of breath. ECG shows sinus bradycardia of 45 beats/min.

197) A 55-year-old woman is noted to have a slow heart rate. She is asymptomatic. ECG shows no relationship between atrial and ventricular rhythm. The ventricular rhythm is 40 beats/min. The QRS complex is wide.

198) A 60-year-old man collapses in the street. The event is unwitnessed. He has no pulse.

199) A 30-year-old man involved in a high-speed RTA is found unconscious at the scene. He is breathing spontaneously. In A&E, the ECG monitor now shows an irregular rhythm and no P, QRS, ST or T waves. The rate is rapid.

200) A 50-year-old man presents to A&E with severe chest pain. He has a history of angina. The pain is not relieved with GTN. BP is 120/70 with a pulse rate of 100. ECG shows regular sinus rhythm.

I. Medicine: SBA/BOF Answers

1) e.
Wegener's granulomatosis is an autoimmune vasculitis that produces
necrotizing granulomas in affected organs. The disease mainly affects the
upper and lower respiratory tracts and the kidneys. Elevation in BP and
abnormal urine results are due to inflamed blood vessels within the
glomeruli. Granulomas located in the lung tissue cause dyspnoea.
Amyloidosis is diagnosed on tissue biopsy.

2) c.
PEA is associated with hypothermia and not with hyperthermia.

3) d.
Malignant otitis externa mainly occurs in immunosuppressed patients
particularly in elderly people with diabetes. It is a complication of simple
otitis externa; the infection (usually *Pseudomonas aeruginosa*) invades
the floor of the ear canal, the surrounding soft tissues and later into the
skull base. Osteomyelitis of the skull base can lead to involvement of
the facial and vagus cranial nerves. Granulation tissue can be seen to line
the floor of the ear canal.

4) a.
Microscopy, culture and sensitivity (MC&S) can be sent to the
laboratory to determine the organism type if an initial dipstick indicates
an infection.

5) c.
The rash is erysipelas – an acute infection of the superficial layers of the
skin. Clinically it resembles cellulitis; however, cellulitis also affects the
deeper subcutaneous layers. Erysipelas is more commonly found in
areas where there is little subcutaneous fat such as the head and face.
Group A streptococci account for over 80% of cases of erysipelas.

6) c.

7) c.
Narrowing of the aorta, usually just distal to the left subclavian artery,
results in aortic coarctation. Typically blood pressures in the right arm
are higher than those in the left, and due to low pressures extremities
remain cold. Takayasu's arteritis tends to occur more often in young
Asian women; peripheral pulses can be difficult to detect due to vascular
narrowings. Kawasaki's disease affects young children presenting with

fever, conjunctivitis, enlarged lymph nodes, and desquamation of the palms and soles. Marfan's syndrome is associated with aortic dissection and aortic dilatation.

8) e.
Certain allergens in sensitized individuals cause a hypersensitivity pneumonitis also known as extrinsic allergic alveolitis (EAA). There are a number of subtypes of EAA including; farmers' lung caused by *Actinomycetes* sp. in mouldy hay, bird-fanciers' lung caused by proteins in bird droppings and cheese-workers' lung caused by the fungus *Penicillium* sp. in cheese mould. Cryptogenic fibrosing alveolitis, as the name suggests, has no known cause.

9) a.
This patient has primary biliary cirrhosis (PBC), an autoimmune disease causing destruction and scarring of the bile canaliculi. Anti-mitochondrial antibodies are found in 95% of cases of PBC and are almost always associated with this condition. Antinuclear antibodies are associated with systemic lupus erythematosus (SLE) but it is a less specific test, as they occur in other autoimmune diseases such as rheumatoid arthritis. Anti-smooth muscle antibodies are associated with chronic active hepatitis.

10) c.
The temporal artery is the most common blood vessel to become affected in cranial arteritis. Inflammation in the branches of this artery reduces blood supply, leading to symptoms such as jaw claudication and visual loss.

11) e.
This is a common condition occurring in children and is caused by overuse of the quadriceps tendon.

12) a.
The common peroneal nerve is at risk with a fracture of the proximal neck of the fibula. It results in foot drop.

13) b.
This patient is having a severe asthma attack. Hydrocortisone, used to dampen inflammation, takes a number of hours to show an effect. Endotracheal intubation will be required if the patient shows no response to initial management or develops life-threatening features.

14) d.
Due to this patient's severe facial injuries and possible damage to the cervical spine, oral and nasal intubations are unfeasible. Cricothyroidotomy is the best intervention that does not require manipulation of the neck.

15) d.
Pulsus parvus et tardus is associated with aortic stenosis.

16) c.

17) e.
VDRL stands for Venereal Disease Research Laboratory test and is used as a screening test for syphilis.

18) b.
The patient has a subdural haematoma. Other patient groups at risk of this type of head injury include people with alcohol problems and elderly patients.

19) c.
The patient has Kaposi's sarcoma, one of the AIDS-defining illnesses.

20) a.
Coeliac disease is associated with folate and iron deficiency.

21) e.
This syndrome is caused by thiamine deficiency.

22) b.
The patient has psoriatic arthritis. Methotrexate, an immuno-suppressant, is a second-line agent and should be considered if non-steroidal anti-inflammatory drugs (NSAIDs) and steroid injections are ineffective.

23) b.
Oxygen, morphine, nitrates and aspirin form the immediate management of a patient with acute coronary syndrome.

24) b.
Atropine helps to improve conduction through the atrioventricular (AV) node by improving sinus node automaticity. Pacing should then be considered urgently.

25) a.
Reversible causes to be evaluated are the 5 Ts (tension pneumothorax, tamponade, toxins, thrombus – coronary, thrombus – pulmonary) and the 5 Hs (hypovolaemia, hypothermia, hyper-/hypokalaemia, hypoxia, hydrogen ions).

26) d.
Also known as Zenker's diverticulum, the pouch forms as a result of herniation of the pharyngeal mucosa posteriorly through Killian's dehiscence.

27) b.
Erythromycin inhibits the hepatic metabolism of carbamazepine, therefore causing toxicity.

28) e.
Papillary carcinomas of the thyroid are well-differentiated cancers and are managed with surgery and radioiodine ablation.

29) a.
Glossitis can be found in folate, vitamin B_{12} and iron deficiency. Hypersegmented neutrophils are, however, pathognomonic of megaloblastic anaemia. Sensory disturbances are due to peripheral nerve demyelination.

30) b.

31) b.
The most common ECG abnormality seen in PE is a tachycardia.

32) a.
β Blockers can mask the symptoms of a hypoglycaemic episode by reducing the development of tremors and palpitations.

33) a.
This patient has CREST syndrome – a subtype of systemic sclerosis. CREST is an acronym for the five main features: Calcinosis, Raynaud's syndrome, Esophageal dysmotility, Sclerodactyly, Telangiectasia.

34) d.
Carcinoid tumours are tumours of the neuroendocrine system and characterized by the production of serotonin.

35) c.

36) c.
This patient has an intracerebral bleed. This patient may also show signs of Cushing's triad: a rising blood pressure, widened pulse pressure and bradycardia – a sign of rising intracranial pressure.

37) c.
The Grey Turner sign is associated with acute pancreatitis.

38) e.
Most allergic conjunctivitis is caused by pollen and antihistamine eye drops will help to ease the symptoms.

39) d.

40) c.
When test results are inconclusive on the diagnosis of diabetes, an oral glucose tolerance test (OGTT) is conducted. A venous glucose plasma level >11.1 mmol/L on an OGTT is diagnostic of diabetes.

41) c.
This patient has infectious mononucleosis.

42) c.
The patient's symptoms, low platelet count and prolonged bleeding time suggest ITP. It is thought to be an autoimmune disease, which runs a chronic course in adults. TTP is a more serious condition presenting with haemolytic anaemia, CNS deficits and renal impairment.

43) c.
This patient has signs of chronic liver disease; the darkened skin pigmentation suggests possible haemochromatosis. Definitive diagnosis is made on liver biopsy.

44) c.

45) c.

46) c.
This is an atypical pneumonia. Hospital outbreaks are not uncommon, hot water being the source of contamination.

47) b.
Extrapyramidal side effects are less common with newer atypical antipsychotics compared with the older typical antipsychotics such as chlorpromazine.

48) e.
The patient has vitamin B_{12} deficiency, causing degeneration of the posterior and lateral columns of the spinal cord.

49) d.

Acral lentiginous melanoma is a type of melanoma seen on the soles and palms, and under the nails. It is the most common type of melanoma in people who are not white.

50) b.

This syndrome consists of ascites, pleural effusion and a benign ovarian tumour.

51) d.

Of patients diagnosed with testicular cancer 10% describe a recent traumatic event to the testicle. The trauma itself does not cause the cancer, but prompts the patient to examine himself and therefore find the abnormality.

52) a.

Thiazides reduce the renal clearance of lithium, resulting in lithium toxicity.

53) d.

Also known as lateral medullary syndrome.

54) c.

This is caused by *Clostridium difficile*. Antibiotic usage from osteomyelitis treatment has changed the gut flora, causing overgrowth of this organism.

55) d.

This patient is having an anaphylactic shock caused by an allergy to penicillin.

56) c.

This should be tried for the first few months and, if ineffective, medication should be started.

57) c.

ACE inhibitors should be avoided in silent atherosclerosis, in particular renal artery stenosis, and may precipitate acute renal failure if administered. Every patient should have a U&E blood test 2 weeks after initiation of an ACE inhibitor to check renal function.

58) e.

59) d.

Ménière's disease is thought to occur from a build-up of fluid in the inner ears, which increases and decreases intermittently, resulting in the patient's episodic attacks. Management entails symptomatic treatment.

60) a.
This remains the gold standard, although it is not used routinely. CTPA is used more frequently due to its non-invasive nature; pulmonary arteriography is used in cases where non-invasive tests are inconclusive.

61) a.
Adenosine is absolutely contraindicated in asthma. β Blockers are also contraindicated but, in rare instances where there is no alternative, a cardioselective β blocker may be prescribed with extreme caution under specialist supervision.

62) d.
Retinal detachment occurs when there is separation between the neurosensory layer (layer of cones and rods) and the pigment layer of the retina. The cause is usually infiltration of fluid through a break in the neurosensory layer. It is an ocular emergency.

63) d.
This is the most common eye infection in AIDS.

64) a.
Small cell carcinoma of the lung is associated with this paraneoplastic syndrome.

65) e.
Choroiditis is associated with unilateral loss of vision.

66) a.

67) d.
A previous cerebrovascular accident is a relative contraindication to thrombolytic therapy.

68) c.
Amphetamines cause an increased level of dopamine in the brain.

69) d.
Rose spots blanch under pressure.

70) d.
Takayasu's arteritis causes inflammation of the aorta and its branches, and tends to occur more often in young women of Oriental origin. Peripheral pulses can be difficult to detect due to vascular narrowing.

71) a.
The patient has infective endocarditis.

72) a.
This is an ocular emergency and requires intravenous antibiotics and regular examination of the function of the optic nerve. Causes include sinusitis of the ethmoid sinus, local infection and trauma to the eye.

73) c.

74) c.
Cold agglutins are antibodies that bind to red blood cells, particularly at low temperatures, to cause agglutination and haemolysis. They form in a number of conditions, including influenza, lymphoma and malaria.

75) d.
This is an autoimmune condition that is usually triggered by an infection – CMV, *Campylobacter* sp. and Epstein–Barr virus (EBV) have been implicated.

76) d.
The palpable node is known as Virchow's node and can be the first sign of gastric carcinoma. It appears in the left supraclavicular region and is the most superficial node at the point where the thoracic duct (through which most of the abdominal lymph drains) empties into the left subclavian vein.

77) a.

78) b.
Lymph node biopsies are done under general anaesthetic.

79) c.
Analysis of these biopsies will show characteristic malignant cells known as Reed–Sternberg cells. These cells have bilobed nuclei and the appearance of an owl's eye under the microscope.

80) c.
This patient has CREST syndrome.

81) a.
Patients on immunosuppressive therapy are at risk of SCC; regular dermatological examination is recommended.

82) b.

83) d.

84) e.

As with all emergencies, basic life support measures should be initiated first. The Guedel airway is precluded due to the patient's trismus.

85) e.

This is a case of gout precipitated by thiazide diuretics.

86) c.

Pethidine is not prescribed because its use is associated with seizures.

87) d.

This patient has liver failure and is unable to maintain normal glucose levels due to inadequate gluconeogenesis and glycogenesis.

88) e.

Most lumbar disc prolapses occur between the fourth and fifth lumbar vertebrae. This patient should also be evaluated for symptoms and signs of cauda equina syndrome – compression of the nerve roots below the level of the spinal cord (level L2).

89) c.

The elevated protein count with a normal cell count is a typical CSF finding.

90) d.

Guillan–Barré syndrome is an autoimmune disease that causes demyelination of the peripheral nerves. Nerve conduction studies are prolonged.

91) a.

Recurrent symptoms in this age group require endoscopy to rule out possible malignancy.

92) e.

Patients with this syndrome are males who have an extra X chromosome. They are tall and thin.

93) b.

94) d.

In an upper motor neuron lesion the forehead is spared because there is bilateral innervation, so the patient is able to wrinkle his forehead. The other options listed are conditions that affect the lower motor neuron of the facial nerve.

95) a.

96) b.
This is also known as scrofula; it is a tuberculous infection of the skin and lymph nodes of the neck.

97) d.
With such a low CD4 count, HIV-affected individuals are considered to have AIDS.

98) e.
This Gram-negative, helix-shaped bacterium infects the lining of the stomach and is implicated in duodenal and gastric ulcers as well as stomach cancers.

99) e.
Heparin may be associated with hyperkalaemia but not hypokalaemia.

100) d.

101) b.
ANAs are seen in a number of autoimmune conditions. More specific tests are conducted after a positive result.

102) c.
Seen in liver disease, diabetes, thyroid disorders and epilepsy.

103) a.

104) c.
Signs of a basal skull fracture: CSF otorrhoea or rhinorrhoea, blood from external auditory meatus, postauricular ecchymosis (Battle's sign), periorbital ecchymosis (raccoon's eyes) and cranial nerve injuries.

105) a.

106) b.

107) b.
This patient has primary biliary cirrhosis. Other autoimmune conditions may be seen simultaneously such as thyroid and coeliac disease.

108) b.
Ascorbic acid (vitamin C) is required for collagen synthesis. Collagen is present in bone, capillaries, skin and dentine tissue. Vitamin C deficiency results in gum haemorrhage and loss of teeth, poor wound healing and haemorrhages.

109) b.
This patient has ankylosing spondylitis.

110) a.
This may show the characteristic bamboo spine picture.

111) c.

112) a.
This is highly specific for SLE and is useful in monitoring flare-ups and remissions.

113) c.
In constrictive pericarditis fatigue is related to low cardiac output and the ascites is caused by an elevation in systemic venous pressure. Other symptoms such as orthopnoea and exertional dyspnoea are related to pulmonary congestion.

114) d.
This is also known as reactive arthritis because inflammation of the joints occurs after an infection elsewhere in the body.

115) e.

116) b.
In premenopausal women the most common cause of iron-deficiency anaemia is menorrhagia. In postmenopasual women the most common cause is gastrointestinal blood loss.

117) b.
These cells with bilobed nuclei are also known as Reed–Sternberg cells.

118) e.

119) e.

120) b.
The clinical picture suggests opiate overdose.

121) e.
Bone metastases are usually associated with low albumin and increased alkaline phosphatase.

122) e.

123) b.

124) a.
The cornea stains like a dendritic tree with sharp borders around the ulcer. The ulcer is caused by the herpes simplex virus.

125) c.
During fetal development of the thyroid gland, buds from the foramen caecum migrate to the lower neck. Persistence of any part of this tract can result in a cyst, sinus or fistula.

126) a.

127) b.
Cor pulmonale describes right heart failure secondary to lung disease. Normal pulmonary artery pressure is approximately 15 mmHg and arterial pressures in cor pulmonale are about 25 mmHg.

128) b.
ECG changes in cor pulmonale include P pulmonale, right axis deviation (RAD), right ventricular hypertrophy (RVH) and inverted T waves in V1–4. The chest radiograph and arterial blood gases may be normal. Lung function tests will show airflow restriction.

129) a.

130) c.

131) d.
Intramuscular diclofenac is the first choice of analgesia; opioids can be administered next if required.

132) c.
Most of the stones that cause renal colic are calcium rich and show up as radio-opaque on a radiograph.

133) d.
Bacteria implicated in pyelonephritis are those of the lower urinary tract: *E. coli*, *Klebsiella* sp., *Proteus* sp.

134) a.
Ectopic pregnancies can be treated surgically with salpingectomy (removal of the fallopian tube containing the ectopic pregnancy) or medically with methotrexate injections.

135) b.

136) b.
This bacterium is able to produce urease, an enzyme that hydrolyses urea to ammonia, thereby causing the urine to become more alkaline.

137) a.

138) b.
Needle cricothyroidotomy may be necessary as an emergency procedure in A&E. The leading cause of death from glandular fever (infectious mononucleosis) is failed endotracheal intubation! Bear in mind that the patient has jaw trismus! Needle cricothyroidotomy will buy time for tracheostomy by an ENT surgeon in theatre.

139) a.

140) b.
This is a reversible acetylcholinesterase inhibitor that increases central levels of acetylcholine and is used in the treatment of Alzheimer's disease.

141) e.
Charcot's joints are also known as neuropathic joints. The joints are severely damaged and disrupted which occurs as a result of loss of sensation in the joint. The most common cause of Charcot's joints is diabetes.

142) c.
Aspiration of the pleural effusion will provide symptomatic relief for the patient as well as allowing investigations of the fluid obtained.

143) b.

An ascitic tap can be used for diagnostic and therapeutic indications.

144) b.

145) a.

Neisseria gonorrhoeae affects columnar epithelium. The vagina is composed of squamous epithelium. This explains why the endocervix and not the vagina is swabbed for the presence of the organism.

146) b.

Oxalate stones are common in Crohn's disease; this patient also consumes a diet high in this salt. In Crohn's disease, fat malabsorption leads to high levels of fatty acids within the colon; these bind to calcium ions leaving high levels of oxalate ions available for absorption (instead of being excreted in the faeces). Hyperoxaluria occurs and crystallization causes stone formation.

147) d.

148) b.

This is a case of spontaneous bacterial peritonitis.

149) e.

Only an upright chest radiograph will show air under the diaphragm.

150) a.

This is a dermatological emergency.

151) a.

The patient exhibits Charcot's triad.

152) b.

153) c.

Penicillamine is a form of treatment for rheumatoid arthritis.

154) c.

155) b.

156) b.
This patient has renal failure. Burr cells can be seen in uraemia.

157) d.
Cystic fibrosis is associated with chronic infection with *Pseudomonas aeruginosa*.

158) b.

159) b.
High titres of dsDNA are almost exclusive to SLE. Only 80% of patients are ANA positive.

160) c.

161) b.
This is an α-haemolytic streptococcus − when grown on blood agar plates it haemolyses the agar substance, causing a green colour change on the plates.

162) b.
The palmar macules described are Janeway's lesions.

163) e.

164) b.
This organism is found in soil and in the normal gastrointestinal flora. Exotoxins released cause muscle necrosis and sepsis.

165) d.

166) e.
Risk factors for bladder cancer include smoking, occupational carcinogens such as arylamines (dye workers/rubber workers) and women receiving radiation treatment for cervical cancer.

167) a.
The trauma has prompted the patient to seek medical attention. Examination suggests a testicular cancer.

168) e.
Although the exact cause of polycystic ovarian syndrome (PCOS) is still not known, insulin resistance has been implicated as a possible factor.

Higher levels of circulating insulin cause more testosterone to be produced from the ovaries than is normal, leading to symptoms of PCOS.

169) d.
Interferon-α is used as part of some cancer treatments such as melanomas and leukaemias. It is also used in the treatment of chronic hepatitis B and C.

170) e.
The repeated cycle of ulceration, alternating with the deposition of granulation tissue during the healing phase, results in the development of raised areas of inflamed tissue, which resemble polyps.

171) a.
Excessive production of aldosterone from an adrenal adenoma is known as Conn's syndrome. Other causes of excessive aldosterone production include adrenal hyperplasia, adrenal carcinoma and renal artery stenosis.

172) a.

173) d.
Peptic ulcer disease is associated with hypercalcaemia not hypocalcaemia.

174) b.
The ulcer erodes into the gastroduodenal artery, which lies behind the superior part of the duodenum, and can cause massive gastrointestinal bleeding.

175) a.

176) a.
Erythromycin is the recommended antibiotic for *Legionella* sp.

177) a.
Hypothyroidism, not hyperthyroidism, is associated with impotence.

178) b.
Staphylococcus aureus is the organism responsible for toxic shock syndrome.

179) a.

180) e.

181) c.
If biopsy is positive for malignancy, further investigation to evaluate the extent of spread is required.

182) b.
There is no history of an upper respiratory tract infection to link to acute vestibular neuronitis.

183) d.
CMV is known to be an immunomodulator and increases the risk of opportunistic infections in immunocompromised patients.

184) c.

185) b.

186) c.
This investigation is highly diagnostic for parathyroid adenomas and for preoperative localization of the parathyroid glands.

187) b.
As in this case, most patients do not have symptoms of Paget's disease. Possible symptoms include pain, bone deformities leading to fractures and nerve compression. Heart failure, bone malignancy and the 'vascular steal syndrome' are rare complications.

188) d.

189) d.
Alcoholism is more associated with vitamin B_1 (thiamine) and folate deficiency. Here gastrectomy is the cause of the vitamin B_{12} deficiency.

190) b.
Tricyclic antidepressant overdose is associated with fits, arrhythmias, urinary retention and pupillary dilatation. Barbiturate poisoning is also associated with pupillary dilatation but not with arrhythmias.

191) a.

192) b.
This is acute respiratory alkalosis induced by a panic attack.

193) c.
This patient has developed a tension pneumothorax and requires immediate needle decompression.

194) d.

195) d.
Hyperglycaemia is a known side effect.

196) c.
Methyldopa is the first-line treatment for hypertension in pregnancy. Second-line treatments include labetalol and nifedipine. Emergency treatment involves intravenous hydralazine. Magnesium sulphate is recommended for the prevention and treatment of seizures.

197) b.

198) a.
Toxoplasma gondii is an obligate intracellular protozoan and causes toxoplasmosis. Toxoplasmosis is one of the AIDS-defining illnesses and in 5% of people with HIV it is the presenting symptom of AIDS.

199) d.

200) b.
The most common bacterium implicated is *Haemophilus influenzae* type b (Hib); the advent of immunization at 2, 3 and 4 months of age has reduced the incidence of epiglottitis.

201) c.
Pulseless ventricular tachycardia is a shockable rhythm.

202) b.
This allows evaluation of the structure and motility function of the oesophagus.

203) e.
Eaton–Lambert syndrome is associated with small-cell carcinoma of the bronchus.

204) b.

205) b.

206) c.
This is the alternative anticoagulant for this patient; the other options are procoagulants.

207) d.
Patients with bulimia have irregular periods. Patients with anorexia have no periods.

208) d.

209) d.
Over 60% of new-onset seizures in this age group are caused by a cerebrovascular accident.

210) d.
This patient presents with classic symptoms and signs of hyperthyroidism.

211) c.

212) d.
Antinuclear antibodies are positive, which is associated with the development of iritis and may lead ultimately to blindness.

213) d.
This patient has polycystic kidney disease. There are three types of this condition: autosomal dominant (as in this patient), autosomal recessive and non-hereditary polycystic kidney disease.

214) e.

215) e.
Post-splenectomy may be associated with early thrombocytosis.

216) a.
The patient needs to be sedated before synchronized cardioversion and specialist help is required.

217) a.
Lobar pneumonia affects a whole lobe of the lung as opposed to bronchopneumonia, which has a more patchy distribution over several lobes.

218) c.

219) b.
Approximately 1 in 12 women of childbearing age has polycystic ovarian syndrome.

220) a.
As the patient is asymptomatic, no treatment is advised at this time.

221) c.
Wernicke's encephalopathy is due to thiamine deficiency, which may be seen in people with chronic alcohol problems, malabsorption, severe vomiting or diarrhoea, and in those with a high carbohydrate intake because thiamine is an essential cofactor in converting carbohydrates to fat.

222) b.
Compression of the median nerve leads to symptoms of carpal tunnel syndrome. Treatment is with splinting, NSAIDs, corticosteroid injections and surgical incision to the transverse carpal ligament.

223) c.

224) b.
This patient has a partial nerve III palsy as the pupils are spared.

225) c.
This patient has polycystic kidney disease; cerebral aneurysms are associated with this condition.

226) b.

227) d.

228) b.
This patient has signs and symptoms of carbon dioxide retention. Doxapram is a respiratory stimulant that acts centrally and is administered intravenously.

229) b.
Digoxin toxicity may be precipitated by hypokalaemia. The ECG changes are consistent with hypokalaemia.

230) c.
Onycholysis refers to the detachment of the nail from its nailbed. This occurs due to a plaque of psoriasis in the distal nailbed with accumulation of scales, which lifts up the nail from the nailbed.

231) c.

232) c.
This is due to metastases from the breast carcinoma into the pituitary gland.

233) b.

234) e.
This is a degenerative disorder of the central and autonomic nervous systems. It was formerly known as Shy–Drager syndrome. Two types exist: MSA-P if parkinsonian symptoms dominate and MSA-C if cerebellar symptoms dominate.

235) b.
The absence of carcinogenic substances and the ill-defined lump point towards a pharyngeal pouch.

236) e.

237) c.
Lead poisoning usually builds up over time and affects a number of systems. Wrist drop is the most common peripheral neuropathy. Burton's line, a blue line across the gums, can also be seen in toxicity.

238) c.

239) b.
Although technically the patient has veno-occlusive disease secondary to bush tea (Jamaican herbal tea) containing pyrrolidizine alkaloids, this condition resembles Budd–Chiari syndrome.

240) a.

241) b.
Cannabis is detectable in urine for up to 27 days with chronic use and for years if a sample of hair is analysed.

242) e.
Obstructive sleep apnoea is associated with carbon dioxide retention and may manifest as morning headaches.

243) b.

244) c.
The cervical spinal cord is most likely to have become compressed by the fall. Cauda equina syndrome presents with perineal numbness, bowel and urinary disorders, low back pain and lower limb weakness.

245) e.

246) a.

247) a.
The sudden increase in intraocular pressure is due to a block in the trabecular meshwork.

248) d.
Vitamin B_1 is also known as thiamine.

249) e.
Streptococcus pneumoniae meningitis is more common among elderly people.

250) c.

251) b.

252) a.

253) a.
This is a long-acting calcium channel blocker. The drug blocks the entry of calcium into the smooth muscle of artery walls, which causes reduced tension in the arterial walls.

254) c.

255) b.
Antifungal therapy consists of topical applications (lozenges, gel or drops) or antifungal tablets.

256) d.
Ankylosing spondylitis is associated with both aortic regurgitation and pulmonary fibrosis. A radiograph of the spine should show squaring of the vertebrae and a characteristic bamboo spine.

257) c.

258) a.

259) b.

260) d.
Enalapril is an ACE (angiotensin-converting enzyme) inhibitor and reduces angiotensin levels.

261) a.
Pleural plaques are associated with asbestosis. Lung function tests will confirm restrictive lung disease.

262) a.
There is no cure; however, corticosteroids are offered. Asbestosis is a risk factor for bronchial carcinoma.

263) d.

264) d.
Heminevrin (chlormethiazole) is no longer recommended for alcohol detoxification because it has been associated with fatalities when

taken together with alcohol. Acamprosate may be offered if a patient requests help in alcohol abstinence after detoxification. Diazepam is the drug of choice for alcohol detoxification.

265) e.

266) e.
Options a–d are standard advice for patients with epilepsy.

267) e.

268) e.

269) e.
Triple therapy is indicated only after confirmation of the presence of *Helicobacter pylori*.

270) a.

271) b.

272) b.
Postoperative arthritis is usually due to gout.

273) a.

274) a.

275) c.

276) e.
Hypoglycaemia is associated with transient loss of consciousness and is reversed immediately with 50% dextrose, 50 mL i.v.

277) c.

278) c.

279) d.

280) b.
According to both the British Hypertension Society and the British Cardiac Society, the 10-year risk of coronary heart disease is based on blood pressure ± diabetes, smoking and cholesterol levels and NOT alcohol consumption.

281) b.
A large proportion of these cases are hereditary and genetic counselling will be required.

282) b.
In a dehydrated patient, early pneumonia will not show up on a chest radiograph! Following rehydration, the pulmonary infiltrate will be more apparent.

283) e.

284) a.
This patient has signs of impending uncal herniation. Seek a neurosurgical consult for possible burr holes.

285) b.
This patient has metastatic breast carcinoma and presents in hypercalcaemic coma.

286) c.

287) a.
Beck's triad reflects the signs of acute cardiac tamponade.

288) a.
A bite from a tick infected with the bacterium *Borrelia* sp. can cause Lyme disease. The rash that appears at the site looks like a 'bull's eye'.

289) a.

290) e.
Surgical resection is the treatment of choice because chemotherapy has not proved to be effective.

291) d.

292) c.
This patient presents with a postoperative haematoma that needs urgent drainage, as it is now compressing her trachea.

293) d.
This is a feature of ulcerative colitis.

294) b.

295) e.
Subcutaneous fragmin twice daily is used as prophylaxis and not treatment of DVT.

296) a.
The four Ts of anterior mediastinal masses are: teratoma, tumour, thyroid mass (goitre or neoplasm), T lymphomas.

297) a.

298) d.

299) d.
Causes of mitral stenosis include rheumatic fever, calcification, endocarditits and congenital disorders.

300) a.
Adenosine slows down electrical impulses through the AV node and therefore, in SVT, allows analysis of the underlying rhythm.

I. Medicine: EMQ Answers

1) **G.**
This tumour marker is a protein that is produced by the cells of the prostate gland.

2) **J.**
Medullary cancer of the thyroid originates from the parafollicular cells of the thyroid (also known as C cells). These cells produce calcitonin.

3) **A.**

4) **K.**
Over 80% of ovarian cancers are surface epithelial cancers; the rest are germ cell tumours.

5) **D.**

6) **A.**
Inability of the lower oesophageal sphincter to relax causes the symptoms in achalasia. A barium swallow is the initial investigation and shows a characteristic bird's beak appearance.

7) **J.**
Battery fluids, drain cleaners and other household cleaning items are commonly used in scenarios such as this one. Alkali ingestions are more damaging than acid ingestions.

8) **E.**

9) **B.**
Pharyngeal pouches are common in the elderly population and are more common in males.

10) **F.**
Most oesophageal cancers are adenocarcinomas or squamous cell carcinomas. Adenocarcinomas occur in the lower third of the oesophagus whereas squamous cell carcinomas occur in the upper parts of the oesophagus.

11) K.
This patient has Addison's disease.

12) G.
This patient presents with classic signs and symptoms of hyperthyroidism.

13) A.
Viable protozoon cysts are ingested in contaminated food.

14) H.
This patient presents with pancreatic cancer. Sudden onset in an elderly patient may be suspicious for pancreatic cancer.

15) I.
Barium swallow followed by upper gastrointestinal endoscopy is needed to exclude oesophageal pathology.

16) H.
Infectious mononucleosis is associated with hepatitis.

17) I.
This is a case of subacute bacterial endocarditis.

18) D.
Unilateral enlargement of the tonsil may be associated with quinsy, lymphoma or carcinoma. Fluctuating fever and the absence of pain suggest a diagnosis of lymphoma.

19) J.
Typical features of sarcoidosis for which Kveim's test is diagnostic.

20) G.
Scrofula is a sign of tuberculosis, for which the Mantoux text is diagnostic.

21) H.
Children aged under 5 years are at risk, because they do not develop specific antibodies against *Haemophilus influenzae* until after the age of 5.

22) D.
Tuberculous meningitis.

23) A.
Meningococcal meningitis.

51) K.
The T-wave changes in V5 and V6 suggest a lateral component to the inferior MI.

52) C.
Atrial fibrillation may be associated with hyperthyroidism.

53) F.

54) H.
Hypokalaemia is a recognized complication of diuretic use.

55) G.

56) B.
The most common cause of Cushing's syndrome is a pituitary adenoma, which is removed via trans-sphenoidal surgery.

57) G.
The pituitary adenoma producing excessive growth hormone is also removed via trans-sphenoidal surgery.

58) A.

59) C.
This patient has multiple endocrine neoplasia (MEN) type II.

60) F.

61) C.
Diabetes mellitus is the most common cause of peripheral neuropathy in the developed world. Glycaemic control is key to the prevention and treatment of diabetic neuropathy.

62) E.
Thiamine deficiency is common in people with alcohol dependence.

63) B.
Chemotherapy agents such as vincristine and cisplatin can cause direct damage to the peripheral nerves.

64) I.

65) G.

66) C.
Cold haemagglutinins are associated with 50% of untreated *Mycoplasma pneumoniae* infection and a titre of 1:64 supports the diagnosis.

67) J.

68) A.

69) B.

70) F.

71) K.
Weight loss and salt restriction are advocated initially.

72) A.

73) B.
As this patient has asthma, β blocker therapy is contraindicated.

74) I.

75) E.

76) J.
Leptospirosis (Weil's disease) is caused by a spirochaete transmitted in water infected by rat urine.

77) F.
Kala-azar or leishmaniasis is spread through the lymphatics via a cutaneous lesion.

78) G.

79) B.

80) I.
Felty's syndrome is the triad of rheumatoid arthritis, splenomegaly and leucopenia.

81) K.
Synthesis of heme, an important constituent of haemoglobin, occurs in the liver. The process is complex in which a large number of enzymes are needed at each step to convert haem precursors (known as porphyrins) into haem itself. Enzyme deficiency can occur at any step of the process leading to accumulation of porphyrins and to symptoms of porphyria. Porphyria is in fact a group of disorders which includes acute intermittent porphyria, cutaneous porphyria and mixed porphyria. Drugs, particularly those containing hormones (e.g. the pill or HRT), infections, smoking and alcohol are known precipitants.

82) F.
Risk factors for renal carcinoma include male gender, age greater than 60 years, workplace carcinogens such as asbestos, high blood pressure and obesity. A right varicocele may develop because the right testicular vein drains into the inferior vena cava (IVC) directly and occlusion of the IVC by a renal mass will cause reduction in blood flow from the testicular arteries into the IVC, and therefore produce a varicocele.

83) B.
IV antibiotics are indicated. Complications of pyelonephritis include septicaemia, renal abscess and premature labour.

84) A.
Ureteric pain is not related to the size of the stone, since even the smallest stone can cause excruciating pain.

85) D.
Acute cystitis (inflammation of the bladder) is usually caused by an infection of the lower urinary tract. *E. coli* is the most common bacterial pathogen.

86) A.
Hypokalaemia is associated with the use of loop diuretics.

87) H.
Convex elevation is suggestive of MI. Here the elevation is concave, which is associated with pericarditis.

88) G.
A diagnosis of inferior MI requires a Q wave in lead II also.

89) C.
Hypocalcaemia is a recognized complication of thyroidectomy.

90) J.
Classic for myxoedema.

91) J.
Anaphylaxis is treated with a prompt injection of 1 mL 1:1000 adrenaline i.m. This may need to be repeated.

92) C.
Tension pneumothorax requires emergency needle decompression.

93) D.
Cardiac tamponade requires swift needle pericardiocentesis.

94) H.
This woman presents with a postoperative haematoma that needs urgent drainage because it is now compressing her trachea.

95) I.
This woman is at risk for a deep vein thrombosis (DVT) and pulmonary embolism (PE). Occasionally the signs of DVT appear after the PE, which can make diagnosis difficult.

96) J.
α_1-Antitrypsin deficiency is often associated with emphysema and liver disease. Liver biopsy gives a definitive diagnosis.

97) A.
Primary biliary cirrhosis is associated with hepatomegaly and a high alkaline phosphatase. Antibodies to mitochondria (AMAs) are found in 95% of cases.

98) B.
The classic triad for idiopathic haemochromatosis is bronze skin pigmentation, diabetes mellitus and hepatomegaly.

99) C.
Kaiser–Fleischer rings are a specific sign for Wilson's disease, a rare inborn error of copper metabolism that leads to a failure of copper excretion.

100) G.
This combination of autoimmune disease and hepatitis is suggestive of autoimmune chronic active hepatitis.

101) H.
Acute lumbar disc prolapse occurs most commonly at L5–S1.

102) J.
Spinal stenosis is treated by surgical decompression.

103) A.
Multiple myeloma is suggestive with a high ESR. Diagnosis is confirmed by the presence of paraprotein in the serum, Bence-Jones protein in the urine and lytic bone lesions.

104) K.
Complications of Paget's disease include deafness, high-output cardiac failure and osteogenic sarcoma.

105) D.
Fusion of the sacroiliac joints is a common feature of ankylosing spondylitis.

106) F.
This is a case of lower motor neuron bladder neuropathy.

107) A.
Excretion urography is useful to investigate the presence of renal disease predisposing to recurrent calculi formation.

108) C.
Dynamic scintigraphy is used to assess renal blood flow, and in this case it is used to establish the extent of renal perfusion post-transplantation.

109) A.
An intravenous urogram will give evidence of renal function in benign prostatic hypertrophy. It may show hydronephrosis, bladder enlargement with chronic retention or intravesical enlargement of the prostate.

110) A.
In retroperitoneal fibrosis, excretion urography allows demonstration of obstruction to the ureter starting at the level of the pelvic brim. Retroperitoneal fibrosis may be associated with retroperitoneal lymphoma, abdominal aortic aneurysm, and carcinoma of the bladder and colon.

111) D.
Bouchard's nodes and 'poor man's gout' are signs of osteoarthritis.

112) G.

113) H.

114) E.

115) A.
Postoperative arthritis is usually due to gout.

116) H.
Right-sided endocarditis is common in intravenous drug users (IVDUs). Other cutaneous lesions of this condition are Osler's nodes (tender nodules on the pulps of fingers and/or toes), Janeway lesions (painless macular purple spots on the palms or soles) and splinter haemorrhages.

117) E.
Drug treatment includes steroids and immunosuppressants, such as azathioprine.

118) F.
If asbestos exposure occurred at the workplace, the patient may be entitled to claim compensation through benefits paid by the government or by suing the employers.

119) J.
This patient has Crohn's disease and a colonoscopy with biopsies are indicated.

120) I.
The leading causes of cirrhosis in the UK are alcoholic liver disease and chronic hepatitis C infection.

121) B.
Management of migraine is divided into treating the acute migraine attack and preventing further episodes from recurring. Acute episodes can be treated with anti-inflammatory analgesics (ibuprofen, diclofenac, naproxen), anti-emetics and triptan-based medications, such as sumatriptan and zolmitriptan. Preventative drugs include propranolol, amitriptyline, pizotifen and some anticonvulsants.

122) C.
Sumatriptan and high-dose oxygen have been found to be very effective in terminating cluster headaches.

123) F.
This boy is suffering from orbital complications of sinusitis and since infection has spread into adjacent structures IV antibiotics are necessary.

124) I.
Management should be initiated immediately to prevent visual loss and high dose oral steroids should be initiated even before a biopsy is performed.

125) G.
Benign intracranial hypertension is seen in obese women of childbearing age. Diplopia results from cranial nerve VI palsy.

126) L.
This is a high risk pregnancy and should be managed under an obstetrician.

127) J.
Most cases are detected within the first year of life. Fallot's teratology is seen in DiGeorge syndrome, an inherited condition, which is implied by the reference to the boy's short stature.

128) K.
Intravenous indomethacin, a prostaglandin inhibitor, is the treatment of choice for patent ductus arteriosus in premature babies.

129) H.
The ECG changes reflect pulmonary hypertension.

130) F.
Tricuspid regurgitation in an intravenous drug user is secondary to infective endocarditis.

131) A.
This is transmitted via inhalation from infected parrots.

132) M.

133) H.

134) I.

135) E.

136) E.
Bilateral internuclear ophthalmoplegia is almost pathognomonic for multiple sclerosis.

137) H.
The Argyll Robertson pupil is almost pathognomonic for neurosyphilis. As her fasting blood glucose is normal, diabetes is excluded as a cause.

138) G.

139) L.

140) K.
Oculomotor nerve lesion with sparing of the pupil is seen with infarction of the oculomotor nerve in diabetes. 'Sparing of the pupil' means that the parasympathetic fibres, which run on the superior surface of the nerve, are spared.

141) B.
Hypoparathyroidism may occur after thyroid or neck surgery.

142) K.

143) I.
This is a case of subdural haemorrhage. Elderly people and people with epilepsy are at risk. Head trauma may have gone unnoticed.

144) L.
The purple papules are most likely Kaposi's sarcoma, associated with HIV.

145) J.
This is a case of hypoglycaemia. Binge drinking and poor nutrition are risk factors.

146) C.

173) F.

174) M.
Travellers' diarrhoea is associated with *Escherichia coli* infection.

175) E.

176) E.
According to the Advanced Trauma Life Support manual published by the American College of Surgeons, until type-specific blood is available (usually takes 10 min and crossmatched blood 1 hour), warmed type O, Rh-negative red blood cells are appropriate in patients with exsanguinating haemorrhage. However, in life-threatening blood loss, the use of unmatched type-specific blood is preferred over type O blood. This patient's chief concern will be massive blood loss. No delay should be taken to crossmatch blood. Blood should be transfused immediately. The blood pressure may be misleading because she is wearing an antishock garment. An external fixator applied by the orthopaedic surgeons will aid in pelvic fracture stabilization and stem blood loss.

177) B.
As both the nasopharynx and oropharynx are compromised, tracheostomy to achieve an airway is essential.

178) C.
With *Haemophilus influenzae* epiglottitis, endotracheal intubation may be difficult. It is necessary to have an ENT surgeon at hand to perform an emergency tracheostomy if the inflamed epiglottis impedes endotracheal intubation.

179) C.
Glandular fever can present as acute airway obstruction. Death from glandular fever occurs from failed endotracheal intubation. It is wise to have an ENT surgeon at hand to perform an emergency tracheostomy if necessary.

180) J.
An acute asthmatic attack is treated initially with oxygen and salbutamol. If necessary intravenous hydrocortisone is added.

181) A.
Children can acquire lead poisoning by eating lead paint chips.

182) D.

183) G.
Cyanide is found in many rodenticides and fertilizers and causes poisoning by inhalation or ingestion.

184) H.
Carbon monoxide poisoning occurs from inadequate ventilation, in this case from the gas fireplace.

185) I.
Insecticides contain inhibitors of cholinesterase and lead to the accumulation of acetylcholine.

186) B.
This is the treatment for hyperglycaemic, hyperosmolar, non-ketotic coma.

187) C.
This is the treatment for diabetic ketoacidosis. The anion gap is 38 mEq/L.

188) E.
Propranolol has been known to induce hypoglycaemia.

189) G.
This patient is most likely septic from a chest infection.

190) H.
This patient has probably self-injected her husband's insulin and has factitious hypoglycaemia.

191) N.
This autoimmune response to a myocardial infarction occurs weeks to months later.

192) C.
In this case, infective endocarditis is the cause of the tricuspid regurgitation.

193) G.
This is an autosomal dominant inherited condition of interventricular septum hypertrophy.

194) D.
Marfan's syndrome is associated with aortic regurgitation.

195) B.
Exertional syncope is a symptom of aortic stenosis. The systolic murmur is classically diamond shaped.

196) A.
Atropine is given to patients with symptomatic bradycardia.

197) E.
Third-degree atrioventricular block is managed with a transvenous pacemaker.

198) C.

199) C.
The patient is in ventricular fibrillation.

200) H.

2. SURGERY

In these questions candidates must select one answer only.

1) A lump is situated above and medial to the pubic tubercle and is felt on the tip of the finger when the patient coughs on scrotal invagination. The most likely diagnosis is:

a. Indirect inguinal hernia
b. Direct inguinal hernia
c. Saphena varix
d. Psoas abscess
e. Femoral hernia

2) A 50-year-old man presents with a groin lump. The lump disappears when the man lies down. He has marked varicose veins. The lump has a fluid thrill. The most likely diagnosis is:

a. Psoas abscess
b. Direct inguinal hernia
c. Saphena varix
d. Femoral artery aneurysm
e. Femoral hernia

3) A 48-year-old woman complains of lower back pain radiating down the buttock, back of thigh and lateral side of the leg to the foot. She also complains of altered perianal sensation and urinary incontinence. The most appropriate management would be:

a. Bedrest
b. Lumbosacral corset
c. Surgical decompression
d. NSAIDs
e. Physiotherapy

4) A 58-year-old man presents with progressive dysphagia to liquids. Of note he has a left recurrent laryngeal nerve palsy. Appropriate management includes all of the following EXCEPT:

a. Chest radiograph
b. LFTs
c. Contrast swallow
d. Upper gastrointestinal (GI) endoscopy and biopsy
e. Total parenteral nutrition

5) Acute pancreatitis may be caused by all of the following EXCEPT:

   a. Diabetes mellitus
   b. Alcoholism
   c. Hyperparathyroidism
   d. Cholelithiasis
   e. Corticosteroids

6) Two days after a right total hip replacement, a 60-year-old obese woman develops shortness of breath. Temperature is 37°C, blood pressure 140/85 and respiratory rate 35/min. On examination she has a swollen right leg. The most likely diagnosis is:

   a. Lymphoedema
   b. Deep venous thrombosis
   c. Pleurisy
   d. Pulmonary embolus
   e. Haematoma

7) Appropriate measures include all of the following EXCEPT:

   a. Intravenous heparin bolus followed by heparin infusion
   b. Subcutaneous fragmin
   c. Oxygen
   d. Pulmonary angiogram
   e. Chest radiograph

8) A 55-year-old man complains of rectal bleeding. He is noted to have freckles on his lips. His father also has freckles on the lips and underwent bowel surgery but he is not sure why. The most likely diagnosis is:

   a. Crohn's disease
   b. Ulcerative colitis
   c. Peutz–Jeghers syndrome
   d. Hereditary haemorrhagic telangiectasia
   e. Familial adenomatous polyposis

9) On preoperative examination, you find a brown, raised, 1-cm lesion on a patient's calf, with irregular borders and ulceration. The next most appropriate step would be:

   a. Palpate the groin for inguinal lymphadenopathy
   b. Take an incisional biopsy of the lesion
   c. Rebook the patient for excisional biopsy
   d. Arrange for a chest radiograph
   e. Notify your senior colleague

10) Calot's triangle is important to visualize in the following surgical procedure:

   a. Abdominal aortic aneurysm repair
   b. Abdominoperineal resection
   c. Mastectomy
   d. Laparoscopic cholecystectomy
   e. Renal transplantation

11) A tall 20-year-old man presents with marked dyspnoea and chest pain. On chest auscultation, there are no breath sounds on the left side, with hyperresonance on percussion. He has just returned from a trans-Atlantic trip to the USA. He is on 100% oxygen and is turning blue. The most likely diagnosis is:

   a. Subcutaneous emphysema
   b. Tension pneumothorax
   c. Pulmonary embolus
   d. *Bacillus anthracis*
   e. Status asthmaticus

12) The most appropriate management would be:

   a. Obtain a chest radiograph
   b. Insert an intercostal chest tube and attach to underwater seal
   c. Intravenous heparinization
   d. Administer ciprofloxacin i.v.
   e. Needle decompression

13) A 40-year-old man presents with haematemesis. He smells of alcohol. After resuscitation with oxygen, intravenous fluids and blood products, what is the next most important step in management?

   a. Contrast swallow
   b. Upper GI series
   c. Endoscopy
   d. Blood for LFTs
   e. Chest radiograph

14) A 30-year-old man presents with a painless swollen right testicle. Appropriate management would include all of the following EXCEPT:

   a. Blood for hCG and α-fetoprotein
   b. Scrotal ultrasonography
   c. CT scan of the abdomen
   d. Chest radiograph
   e. A 12-lead ECG

15) A 36-year-old woman presents with cyclical bilateral breast pain. Appropriate management after excluding sinister causes includes all of the following EXCEPT:

a. Evening primrose oil
b. Oral contraceptive pill
c. Danazol
d. Gamolenic acid
e. Bromocriptine

16) A 32-year-old woman presents with a right breast lump and right breast pain. On examination she has a tender 1-cm breast lump. The most appropriate management in the clinic would be:

a. Fine-needle aspiration
b. Ultrasonography of the breasts
c. Mammogram
d. Tru-Cut biopsy
e. List for excisional biopsy

17) A 40-year-old man on high-dose steroids and azathioprine for acute exacerbation of his Crohn's disease now presents with severe upper abdominal pain and vomiting. The most likely diagnosis is:

a. Small bowel obstruction
b. Perforated peptic ulcer
c. Acute cholecystitis
d. Toxic megacolon
e. Ischaemic colitis

18) The most useful initial investigation would be:

a. Upright chest radiograph
b. Abdominal radiograph
c. Endoscopy
d. Contrast swallow
e. Abdominal ultrasonography

19) A mammogram shows microcalcifications. The most appropriate management would be:

a. Repeat mammogram immediately
b. Breast ultrasonography
c. Needle-guided breast biopsy
d. Nil
e. Repeat mammogram in 1 year

20) Two days after coronary artery bypass graft, a 50-year-old man complains of severe abdominal pain, distension and vomiting. The serum amylase is elevated with high leucocytosis. Plain abdominal radiograph shows an ileus. The most likely diagnosis is:

   a. Acute mesenteric ischaemia
   b. Ruptured abdominal aortic aneurysm
   c. Acute pancreatitis
   d. Perforated peptic ulcer
   e. Small bowel obstruction

21) The definitive investigation to confirm the suspected diagnosis is:

   a. Barium enema
   b. Colonoscopy
   c. Angiography
   d. CT scan of the abdomen
   e. Abdominal ultrasonography

22) A 70-year-old woman falls onto her outstretched hand. A radiograph reveals a proximal humeral fracture. The most likely nerve to be damaged secondary to her fracture is:

   a. Ulnar nerve
   b. Radial nerve
   c. Axillary nerve
   d. Tibial nerve
   e. Median nerve

23) The patient will be unable to carry out the following manoeuvres:

   a. Abduct her shoulder
   b. Supinate her forearm
   c. Pronate her forearm
   d. Make a fist
   e. Adduct her wrist

24) The following statements about the treatment of breast cancer are true EXCEPT:

   a. Locoregional breast cancer may be treated with wide local excision+radiotherapy
   b. Locoregional breast cancer may be treated with mastectomy and radiotherapy to the flaps
   c. If the sentinel node biopsy is positive, proceed to axillary node clearance
   d. Primary chemotherapy may be used to treat inflammatory breast cancer
   e. Postmenopausal women with breast cancer and positive oestrogen receptors should be offered tamoxifen

25) A fine-needle aspirate cytology is sufficient to diagnose all of the following EXCEPT:

a. Papillary thyroid carcinoma
b. Follicular thyroid carcinoma
c. Medullary thyroid carcinoma
d. Anaplastic thyroid carcinoma
e. Lymphoma

26) Complications of steroid therapy include all of the following EXCEPT:

a. Avascular necrosis of the hip
b. Adrenal hyperplasia
c. Peptic ulceration
d. Acute pancreatitis
e. Osteoporosis

27) On routine preoperative examination, a 55-year-old man is found to have a pulsatile midline abdominal mass. The most useful investigation would be:

a. CT scan of the abdomen
b. Digital subtraction angiography
c. Ultrasonography of the abdomen
d. Abdominal radiograph
e. MRI of the abdomen

28) The following statements regarding testicular tumours are correct EXCEPT:

a. Seminomas usually present in men in their 40s
b. Teratomas are radiosensitive
c. Cryptorchism is a risk factor
d. The contralateral testicle should be biopsied, if there is a history of infertility
e. After orchidectomy the disease is staged by chest and abdominal CT scans

29) A parotid mass is most likely to be malignant if the following feature is present:

a. Facial nerve palsy
b. Pain
c. Recent enlargement
d. Foul duct discharge
e. Stenosed ductal meatus

30) A 65-year-old man presents with a 2-month history of vague lower abdominal pain, alternating diarrhoea with constipation and 4-kg weight loss. He has passed a small amount of dark red blood per rectum. There is anaemia. The most likely diagnosis is:

   a. Diverticular disease
   b. Crohn's disease
   c. Ulcerative colitis
   d. Angiodysplasia
   e. Carcinoma of the colon

31) A 65-year-old woman presents with blood per rectum and weight loss. The most useful investigation would be:

   a. Barium enema
   b. Sigmoidoscopy
   c. Colonoscopy
   d. Endoscopy
   e. Proctoscopy

32) A 20-year-old woman presents with a wrist laceration. To test the function of the median nerve, you ask her to:

   a. Extend the thumb
   b. Palmar abduct the thumb against resistance
   c. Pinch paper between the thumb and index finger leading to flexion of the DIP (distal interphalangeal) joint
   d. Extend the fingers completely and spread them apart
   e. Adduct the thumb

33) Charcot's triad is:

   a. Epigastric pain, jaundice and fever with rigors
   b. Enlarged liver, jaundice and fever with rigors
   c. Palpable gallbladder, jaundice and fever with rigors
   d. Fever, right upper quadrant pain and a palpable mass
   e. Fever with rigors, jaundice and right upper quadrant pain

34) Courvoisier's law states that 'if in the presence of jaundice the gallbladder is palpable, then the jaundice is . . .':

   a. Attributable to gallstones
   b. Unlikely to be due to a stone
   c. Likely to be due to a tumour of the head of the pancreas
   d. Due to cholangitis
   e. Likely to be due to carcinoma of the bile duct arising above the origin of the cystic duct

35) What is the first diagnostic test for suspected gallstones?

   a. Serum bilirubin
   b. Abdominal radiograph
   c. Ultrasonography
   d. ERCP (endoscopic retrograde cholangiopancreatography)
   e. HIDA (hepatobiliary iminodiacetic acid) scan

36) The following are causes of acute pancreatitis EXCEPT:

   a. Alcoholism
   b. Biliary tract disease
   c. Oestrogens
   d. Loop diuretics
   e. Mumps

37) Risk factors for DVT include all of the following EXCEPT:

   a. Total hip replacement
   b. Caesarean section
   c. Malignancy
   d. Cardiac failure
   e. Osteoporosis

38) What is the definitive investigation for DVT?

   a. Duplex scanning
   b. Doppler ultrasonography
   c. Venous plethysmography
   d. Venography
   e. Ventilation–perfusion scan

39) What is the most common cause of postoperative renal failure?

   a. Pre-existing renal disease
   b. Hypertension
   c. Renal artery stenosis
   d. Diabetes mellitus
   e. Hypovolaemia

40) A 60-year-old man has a temperature of 38.5°C without rigors 24 hours postoperatively. The most likely cause of the pyrexia is:

   a. DVT
   b. Pneumonia
   c. Thrombophlebitis
   d. Urinary tract infection
   e. Atelectasis

41) A 50-year-old man post-nephrectomy 3 days ago now presents with fever and confusion. On examination there are no breath sounds in the right lung base and no bowel sounds. The most likely diagnosis is:

a. Aspiration pneumonia
b. Pulmonary embolus
c. Atelectasis
d. Pneumonia
e. Pneumothorax

42) A 55-year-old man presents with diarrhoea 3 days after an abdominal aortic aneurysm repair. On examination the abdomen is distended, very tender, with no active bowel sounds. The most likely diagnosis is:

a. Pseudomembranous colitis
b. Mesenteric ischaemia
c. Bowel viscus perforation
d. *Shigella* dysentery
e. Faecal impaction

43) A 30 year old who is a cyclist is involved in an RTA. He sustains multiple injuries and undergoes open reduction and internal fixation of the right femur. On postoperative day 3 he becomes acutely short of breath. The most useful investigation is:

a. Arterial blood gas
b. Chest radiograph
c. FBC
d. Blood cultures
e. A 12-lead ECG

44) The most likely diagnosis is:

a. Acute myocardial infarction
b. Pulmonary embolus
c. Hypovolaemia due to blood loss
d. Septicaemia
e. Chest infection

45) A 60-year-old man is diagnosed with a tumour of the head of the pancreas. The patient should be offered:

a. Distal pancreatectomy
b. Pancreaticojejunostomy
c. Whipple's procedure (pancreaticoduodenectomy)
d. Total pancreatectomy
e. Multiple drug chemotherapy with radiation

46) A 35-year-old woman presents with a 1-month history of a painless firm but mobile 2-cm lump in the upper outer quadrant of her breast. No other abnormalities detected. Initial investigation should be:

a. Mammogram
b. Ultrasonography
c. Fine-needle aspiration cytology
d. Tru-Cut biopsy
e. Assessment for *BRCA*-1 and -2 mutations with sentinel node biopsy

47) The five 'Ps' of arterial insufficiency include all of the following EXCEPT:

a. Pallor
b. Paraesthesia
c. Paralysis
d. Painless
e. Pulseless

48) McBurney's point is located:

a. At the outer third of a line joining the umbilicus to the anterosuperior iliac spine
b. At the outer third of a line joining the umbilicus to the anteroinferior iliac spine
c. At the inner third of a line joining the anterosuperior iliac spine to the pubic tubercle
d. At the inner third of a line joining the umbilicus to the anterosuperior iliac spine
e. At the outer third of a line joining the anterosuperior iliac spine to the pubic tubercle

49) The borders of Hesselbach's triangle include the epigastric vessels, the edge of the rectus sheath and the following structure:

a. Poupart's ligament (the reflected inguinal ligament)
b. The internal oblique aponeurosis
c. The external oblique aponeurosis
d. Transversalis fascia
e. The conjoint tendon

50) A 45-year-old man with a history of ulcerative colitis now presents with nausea, vomiting and abdominal distension. Plain abdominal films show dilatation of the entire colon. The most likely diagnosis is:

a. Volvulus
b. Diverticular disease of the colon
c. Toxic megacolon
d. Paralytic ileus
e. Carcinoma

51) Medical management of ulcerative colitis includes all of the following EXCEPT:

a. Methylcellulose
b. Mesalazine
c. Predsol suppository
d. Azathioprine
e. Loperamide

52) A 20-year-old man presents with a cut over the right metacarpophalangeal joint. Appropriate management includes all of the following EXCEPT:

a. Obtain a hand radiograph
b. Close with sutures using aseptic technique
c. Prescribe broad-spectrum antibiotics
d. Debride and irrigate the wound
e. Swab the wound for culture and sensitivity

53) The following statements about skin carcinoma are true EXCEPT:

a. Basal cell carcinoma rarely metastasizes
b. Squamous cell carcinoma may occur in irradiated tissue
c. Keratoacanthoma is premalignant
d. Squamous cell carcinoma grows more rapidly than basal cell carcinoma
e. Actinic keratoses are premalignant

54) The different types of malignant melanoma include all of the following EXCEPT:

a. Superficial spreading
b. Lentigo maligna
c. Nodular
d. Acral lentiginous
e. Nodular sclerosing

55) A 60-year-old man presents with sudden, severe, colicky pain and bloody diarrhoea that began after lunch 3 hours ago. He has a history of two myocardial infarctions. On examination: temperature 39°C, BP 130/90, pulse 110/min regular. There is rebound tenderness in the lower left quadrant of his abdomen and there is fresh blood present in the rectum. There is a raised white cell count and mild anaemia. The most likely diagnosis is:

a. Colon carcinoma
b. Diverticular disease
c. Inferior mesenteric artery ischaemia
d. Superior mesenteric artery thromboembolism
e. *Campylobacter* infection

56) Treatment options for prostatic adenocarcinomas include all of the following EXCEPT:

   a. Local radiotherapy
   b. Transurethral resection of the prostate (TURP)
   c. Chemotherapy
   d. Cyproterone acetate
   e. Orchidectomy

57) Complications of burns include all of the following EXCEPT:

   a. Stress ulcer
   b. ARDS (acute respiratory distress syndrome)
   c. Adynamic ileus
   d. Sepsis
   e. Hypoglycaemia

58) A 25-year-old woman presents with a 4-year history of intermittent bloody diarrhoea, abdominal pain and fever. Stool cultures are negative. Barium enema studies reveal loss of haustral markings in the colon. Sigmoidoscopy shows an erythematous and friable mucosa. The most likely diagnosis is:

   a. Crohn's disease
   b. Diverticulosis
   c. Peutz–Jeghers syndrome
   d. Shigellosis
   e. Ulcerative colitis

59) A 30-year-old man presents with a crush injury to the right anterior leg. The leg is swollen, painful and pulseless. The most appropriate management would be:

   a. Fasciotomy
   b. Arteriogram
   c. Plain radiograph of the leg
   d. Duplex scanning
   e. Start heparin infusion

60) Indications for carotid endarterectomy include all of the following EXCEPT:

   a. Recurrent transient ischaemic accidents (TIAs)
   b. Non-stenotic atherosclerotic ulcers
   c. Total occlusion of the internal carotid artery
   d. Reduction in diameter of carotid artery by >70%
   e. Symptomless patients with a high-grade stenosis as prophylaxis against stroke before cardiac bypass surgery

61) Malignant melanoma occurring in the following sites are associated with a poorer prognosis stage for stage EXCEPT for:

a. Back
b. Neck
c. Scalp
d. Trunk
e. Leg

62) A 50-year-old man presents with haematuria. MSU reveals a sterile pyuria. This is suggestive of a diagnosis of:

a. Urinary calculi
b. Tuberculosis
c. Glomerulonephritis
d. Hydronephrosis
e. Neoplasm

63) A 55-year-old white man involved in an RTA is found to have blood at the urethral meatus. Management includes all of the following EXCEPT:

a. Retrograde urethrogram
b. Pelvic radiograph
c. Suprapubic catheter
d. Digital rectal examination
e. Foley catheterization

64) Painless haematuria is most likely to be associated with:

a. Urinary tract infection
b. Bladder tumour
c. Gonorrhoea
d. Sickle cell anaemia
e. Renal calculi

65) A 60-year-old woman after right hemicolectomy is found to have glycosuria. This is confirmed by an elevated serum glucose. Possible causes include all of the following EXCEPT:

a. Sepsis
b. Pre-existing diabetes mellitus
c. Parenteral nutrition
d. Concurrent use of steroids
e. Liver failure

66) A 70-year-old woman presents with dysphagia and regurgitation to solids. She also has halitosis. There is a small lump on the left side of her neck. The most appropriate investigation is:

   a. Barium swallow
   b. Oesophagoscopy
   c. Neck radiograph
   d. Neck ultrasonography
   e. Thyroid function tests

67) A 40-year-old woman undergoes rigid oesophagoscopy for the removal of a piece of chicken bone. She now presents with severe chest pain. The most likely diagnosis is:

   a. Acute myocardial infarction
   b. Pulmonary embolus
   c. Oesophageal perforation
   d. Boerhaave's syndrome
   e. Perforated peptic ulcer

68) Diagnosis is best confirmed on:

   a. Plain, soft-tissue, neck radiograph
   b. A 12-lead ECG
   c. Upright chest radiograph
   d. Gastrografin swallow
   e. Barium swallow

69) A 20-year-old woman presents with a 5-day history of right iliac fossa (RIF) pain. On examination a mass is palpated in the RIF. The abdomen is soft with active bowel sounds. Possible causes include all of the following EXCEPT:

   a. Ectopic pregnancy
   b. Appendiceal mass
   c. Acute appendicitis
   d. Ovarian cyst
   e. Crohn's disease

70) A 19-year-old man presents with abdominal pain. On palpation of the left lower quadrant pain is felt in the right lower quadrant. This phenomenon is known as:

   a. Rebound tenderness
   b. Babinski's response
   c. Rovsing's sign
   d. Pemberton's sign
   e. Froment's sign

71) A 70-year-old woman presents with vomiting. On examination there is a tense and tender groin lump present below and lateral to the pubic tubercle. It is not reducible and there is no cough impulse. The most likely diagnosis is:

    a. Strangulated indirect inguinal hernia
    b. Strangulated direct inguinal hernia
    c. Saphena varix
    d. Psoas abscess
    e. Strangulated femoral hernia

72) The most likely hernia to strangulate is:

    a. Umbilical
    b. Indirect
    c. Direct
    d. Femoral
    e. Obturator

73) A 50-year-old obese woman presents with pyrexia, vomiting and upper abdominal pain. On examination there is a palpable mass in the right upper quadrant. The sclerae are white. The most likely diagnosis is:

    a. Biliary colic
    b. Acute cholecystitis
    c. Typhoid fever
    d. Stone in the common bile duct
    e. Hiatus hernia

74) A 50-year-old man post-cholecystectomy now presents with jaundice. He is apyrexial. His urine is dark and his stools are pale. The most likely diagnosis is:

    a. Carcinoma of the head of the pancreas
    b. Mucocele
    c. Common bile duct stone
    d. Primary biliary cirrhosis
    e. Cholangitis

75) The most useful investigation is:

    a. ERCP
    b. Ultrasonography
    c. CT scan
    d. Intravenous cholangiography
    e. Barium meal

76) Perioperative blood transfusion is detrimental in the following condition:

    a. Aortic surgery
    b. Colonic carcinoma
    c. Total hip replacement
    d. Coronary artery bypass graft
    e. Pancreatic carcinoma

77) The following are absorbable sutures EXCEPT:

    a. Catgut
    b. Dexon
    c. Vicryl
    d. PDS
    e. Prolene

78) A 60-year-old man post-TURP presents with convulsions. Blood pressure is 90/50. Laboratory results show hyponatraemia. The most likely complication is:

    a. Clot retention
    b. Haemorrhage
    c. TURP syndrome
    d. ABO incompatibility
    e. ARDS

79) Types of staging include all of the following EXCEPT:

    a. Clinical
    b. Radiological
    c. Surgical
    d. Pathological
    e. Historical

80) Operative treatment for carcinoma of the descending colon is:

    a. Right hemicolectomy
    b. Transverse colectomy
    c. Left hemicolectomy
    d. Hartmann's procedure
    e. Total colectomy

81) Investigations in the assessment of a patient with a history of TIAs include all of the following EXCEPT:

    a. FBC
    b. A 12-lead ECG
    c. CT scan of the head
    d. Carotid digital subtraction angiogram
    e. Positron emission tomography (PET)

82) The most common cause of mechanical small bowel obstruction is:
    a. Crohn's disease
    b. Hernias
    c. Carcinoma
    d. Adhesions
    e. Gallstone ileus

83) A 50-year-old man presents with severe flank pain and haematuria. Appropriate analgesia would be:
    a. Diclofenac
    b. Pethidine
    c. Diamorphine
    d. Co-proxamol
    e. Tramadol

84) An intravenous urogram reveals a 3-cm stone in the left renal pelvis with dilatation of the calyces. Initial treatment would be:
    a. Percutaneous nephrostomy
    b. Extracorporeal shock wave lithotripsy
    c. Nephrolithotomy
    d. Partial nephrectomy
    e. Extraction using a Dormia basket

85) Appropriate prophylactic antibiotic for total hip replacement surgery would be:
    a. Penicillin
    b. Cefuroxime
    c. Metronidazole
    d. Amoxicillin
    e. Flucloxacillin

86) Prophylactic antibiotic of choice for appendectomy is:
    a. Cefuroxime
    b. Penicillin
    c. Metronidazole
    d. Vancomycin
    e. Gentamicin

87) Management for splenectomy patients includes all of the following EXCEPT:
    a. Preoperative Pneumovax
    b. Preoperative meningococcal vaccine
    c. Preoperative Hib vaccine
    d. Life-long amoxicillin
    e. Life-long penicillin

88) Prophylactic antibiotic of choice for cardiac valve replacement operations is:

a. Penicillin
b. Cefuroxime
c. Co-amoxiclav
d. Vancomycin
e. Flucloxacillin

89) Components of an audit cycle include all of the following EXCEPT:

a. Implementing change
b. Selecting a topic
c. Observing practice
d. Comparing practice with standards
e. Managing risk

90) The best investigation of choice for assessing the severity of acute pancreatitis is:

a. Dynamic CT scan
b. Serum amylase
c. Abdominal ultrasonography
d. Urinary amylase
e. ERCP

91) Which specific blood test should be requested for a patient with suspected DVT?

a. FBC
b. PT
c. D-dimers
d. APTT
e. Bleeding time

92) A 75-year-old man presents with urinary retention. On examination he has an enlarged prostate. Blood tests reveal a normal prostate-specific antigen (PSA). Appropriate management includes any of the following EXCEPT:

a. α Blocker
b. TURP
c. Anti-androgen finasteride
d. Antimuscarinic
e. Parasympathomimetic

93) A 10-year-old boy falls off his bicycle and presents with contusion of the right hand. On examination he has a swollen thenar eminence. He is tender in the anatomical snuffbox. He has weakness of opponens pollicis and normal abductor pollicis brevis function. What is your suspected diagnosis?

a. Radial nerve palsy
b. Median nerve palsy
c. Fracture of the scaphoid
d. Colles' fracture
e. Fracture of the metacarpal bone

94) A 22 year old who is an intravenous drug abuser has injected into the anatomical snuffbox and is now unable to extend his wrist. What is his diagnosis?

a. Median nerve palsy
b. Radial nerve palsy
c. Ulnar nerve palsy
d. Scaphoid fracture
e. Colles' fracture

95) A 70-year-old man is noted to have a BP of 170/100. Before starting his medication, the following blood tests should be requested EXCEPT:

a. FBC
b. U&Es
c. Lipids
d. TFTs
e. Clotting screen

96) A 60-year-old man complains of recurrent TIAs. Initial diagnosis is made by:

a. A 12-lead ECG
b. CT scan of the head
c. Intravenous digital subtraction arteriogram of the carotids
d. Duplex scan of the carotids
e. Intra-arterial digital subtraction angiography (IADSA)

97) Complications that can occur with a tracheostomy include all of the following EXCEPT:

a. Tracheal stenosis
b. Posterior wall erosion
c. Displaced tube
d. Acquired tracheo-oesophageal fistula
e. Infection with *Pseudomonas aeruginosa*

98) Complications of massive blood transfusions include all of the following EXCEPT:

a. Depletion of clotting factors
b. Hypocalcaemia
c. Hypothermia
d. Hypokalaemia
e. Thrombocytopenia

99) A 60-year-old man on day 1 postoperatively after a Hartmann's procedure presents with a temperature of 40°C and a BP of 80/50. Urine output is now only 10 mL/h. The most likely diagnosis is:

a. Septicaemic shock
b. Cardiogenic shock
c. Hypovolaemic shock
d. Neurogenic shock
e. Anaphylactic shock

100) Appropriate measures for this man include all of the following EXCEPT:

a. Blood cultures
b. Wound culture
c. Start intravenous cefuroxime and metronidazole
d. Start dopamine
e. Start furosemide

101) Patients who have undergone a gastrectomy may need to take a supplement of the following vitamin:

a. Vitamin K
b. Vitamin B_{12}
c. Vitamin B_6
d. Vitamin C
e. Vitamin E

102) A 49-year-old woman presents with confusion. She is noted to have a serum calcium of 3.2 mmol/L. On examination a 3-cm lump is palpated in her left breast. Management should include the following EXCEPT:

a. Intravenous fluids
b. Oxygen
c. Calcitonin
d. Bisphosphonates
e. Tamoxifen

103) A 55-year-old woman presents with disfiguring varicose veins. She reports that her legs ache by the end of the day. Examination should include all of the following EXCEPT:

   a. Perform Brodie–Trendelenburg tourniquet test
   b. Check for cough impulse over saphenofemoral junction
   c. Percuss over varix
   d. Check peripheral pulses
   e. Inspect for ankle flare and eczema

104) Diagnostic investigations include all of the following EXCEPT:

   a. Doppler ultrasonography
   b. Duplex ultrasonic Doppler scan
   c. Varicography
   d. Radionuclide venography
   e. Bipedal ascending plethysmography

105) A 40-year-old man presents with fever, anal pain and perianal inflammation. On examination you confirm a perianal abscess. The most appropriate management is:

   a. EUA (explore under anaesthetic), investigate and identify (I&D) ± biopsy
   b. Conservative treatment with metronidazole
   c. Bedrest and analgesia
   d. Wide local excision with healing by primary suture
   e. Lateral sphincterotomy

106) Complications of below-knee amputations include all of the following EXCEPT:

   a. Neuroma
   b. Gas gangrene
   c. Osteomyelitis
   d. Contracture
   e. Phantom pain

107) Signs of inoperable breast cancer include all of the following EXCEPT:

   a. Peau d'orange
   b. Skin ulceration
   c. 5-cm breast lump
   d. Satellite nodules
   e. Chest fixity

108) A 55-year-old woman with metastatic breast disease now has a pathological fracture of the right femur. The most appropriate management would be:

    a. Intramedullary nail
    b. Internal fixation with plate and screws
    c. Radiotherapy
    d. Skin traction
    e. Chemotherapy with CMF (cyclophosphamide, methotrexate, 5-fluorouracil)

109) The UK National Breast Screening Programme currently advises mammography every 3 years to women aged between:

    a. 40 and 65
    b. 45 and 64
    c. 50 and 70
    d. 45 and 60
    e. 35 and 59

110) Lateral neck lumps include all of the following EXCEPT:

    a. Cystic hygroma
    b. Branchial cyst
    c. Tuberculous cervical adenitis
    d. Carotid body tumour
    e. Dermoid cyst

111) A 20-year-old man is brought to A&E complaining of headache and drowsiness. On examination he has a boggy swelling over the left side of his skull. The left pupil is dilated and unresponsive to light. The most likely diagnosis is:

    a. Cerebral malignancy
    b. Extradural haemorrhage
    c. Subdural haematoma
    d. Meningitis
    e. Subarachnoid haemorrhage

112) The most common site of diverticulitis in the colon is within the:

    a. Ascending colon
    b. Descending colon
    c. Rectum
    d. Sigmoid
    e. Transverse colon

113) A 17-year-old young man fell on to the crossbar of his bicycle and now complains of pain in his scrotum. On examination he has a haematoma in the perineum and scrotum, and blood from the urethral meatus. He has the urge to urinate but cannot due to pain. He has a palpable bladder. Initial measures may include all of the following EXCEPT:

   a. Broad-spectrum antibiotics
   b. Ascending urethrography using a water-soluble contrast
   c. Passage of a urinary catheter per urethra
   d. Insertion of a suprapubic catheter
   e. Analgesia

114) Of the following list of complications, total hip replacement surgery has the highest risk of:

   a. Death
   b. DVT/PE
   c. Wound infection
   d. Urinary retention
   e. Sciatic nerve damage

115) A 50-year-old man presents with severe abdominal pain radiating to his back. His blood pressure is 80/40 with a pulse rate of 120. The following measures should be taken EXCEPT:

   a. CT scan of the abdomen
   b. A 12-lead ECG
   c. Type and crossmatch 10 units of blood
   d. Give blood or plasma expanders via a central line
   e. Crash induction of anaesthesia in the operating theatre

116) The patient is anaesthetized and on the table. You are a junior doctor on a busy vascular service at a district general hospital and the registrar informs the theatre that he is on his way but is delayed. There is no specialty registrar on duty and the consultant is at home. The anaesthetist is unable to sustain the patient's BP. He tells you to open the patient. You decide to perform a long midline abdominal incision. You confirm a ruptured aortic aneurysm. You could buy time by all of the following EXCEPT:

   a. Put your hand over the hole in the aorta
   b. Place a clamp over the neck of the aneurysm
   c. Insert a large Foley catheter on an introducer through the rupture and inflate the balloon
   d. Place a clamp over the suprarenal aorta
   e. Suction the blood from the abdominal cavity

117) A 35-year-old woman presents with shortness of breath following a subtotal thyroidectomy. Likely causes include all of the following EXCEPT:

a. Laryngeal oedema
b. Haemorrhage into the paratracheal space
c. Aspiration of vomit
d. Unilateral or bilateral vocal fold palsy
e. Pulmonary embolus

118) Likely complications occurring after laparoscopic cholecystectomy include all of the following EXCEPT:

a. Bleeding
b. Jaundice
c. Biliary peritonitis
d. Umbilical hernia
e. Paralytic ileus

119) Initial investigations for jaundice should include all of the following EXCEPT:

a. LFTs
b. Hepatitis A, B and C virology
c. Urine for bilirubin and urobilinogen
d. ERCP
e. EBV and CMV serology

120) What is the best technique for managing retained common bile duct stones?

a. ERCP and sphincterotomy
b. Endoscopic removal or destruction of stones via a T-tube tract
c. Surgical exploration
d. Electrohydraulic or laser lithotripsy
e. Irrigation down a T tube with saline

121) A 22-year-old man presents with a gunshot wound to the right anterior thigh. You are unable to palpate any distal pulses and the leg is cold. You are also unable to detect any pulses by Doppler ultrasound probe. The next step should be:

a. Urgent fasciotomy
b. Urgent arteriography
c. Surgical exploration
d. Radiograph of leg
e. Ascending plethysmography

122) A 55-year-old man presents with having lost a stone over the last 6 months. He has smoked three packs of cigarettes per day over the last 35 years. On examination he has distended neck veins and a puffy face. The most likely cause is:

a. Congestive heart failure
b. Enlargement of bullae
c. Obstruction of the superior vena cava
d. Pulmonary embolus
e. Thrombosis of the subclavian vein

123) Best management for pyloric stenosis is:

a. Hydrostatic reduction by barium enema
b. Ramstedt's pyloromyotomy
c. Duodeno-duodenostomy
d. Exploratory laparotomy
e. Bedrest and intravenous fluids

124) A 16-year-old young man presents with acute onset of severe testicular pain and swelling. There is no history of trauma. The cord is thickened and the testis is tender, hot and swollen. Management should be:

a. Take urethral swabs and MSU
b. Give doxycycline and ciprofloxacin
c. Obtain consent and place on emergency list for possible orchidectomy and bilateral orchidopexy
d. Obtain ultrasonography of the testis
e. Take blood for serum βhCG and α-fetoprotein

125) The surgical procedure of choice for ulcerative colitis is:

a. Hartmann's procedure
b. Panproctocolectomy
c. Subtotal colectomy and RIF end-ileostomy
d. Restorative proctocolectomy
e. Split-loop ileostomy

126) A 70-year-old man presents with profuse per rectum bleeding. He has a history of aortic valve replacement. Management may include all of the following EXCEPT:

a. Colonoscopy
b. Barium enema
c. Radiolabelled red cell scanning
d. Proctoscopy and sigmoidoscopy
e. Selective mesenteric angiography

127) Treatment for angiodysplasia is:

a. Right hemicolectomy
b. Sigmoid colectomy
c. Subtotal colectomy
d. Colonoscopic laser or diathermy
e. Conservative treatment with blood transfusions

128) A 65-year-old woman presents with fever, vomiting and severe left lower abdominal pain. On examination she has rebound tenderness and left iliac fossa guarding. The most appropriate management would be:

a. Intravenous broad-spectrum antibiotics and barium enema
b. Flexible sigmoidoscopy
c. Laparotomy and Hartmann's procedure (subtotal colectomy with ileostomy and closure of the sigmoid colon at the peritoneal reflection)
d. Drainage and proximal loop colostomy
e. Resection with primary anastomosis

129) The correct 5-year survival rate for Dukes' stage B rectal carcinoma is:

a. 68%
b. 50%
c. 40%
d. 26.5%
e. 16.4%

130) Stigmata of liver disease include all of the following EXCEPT:

a. Xanthomas
b. Palmar erythema
c. Gynaecomastia
d. Volkmann's contracture
e. Clubbing

131) Cholangiocarcinoma is associated with which parasite?

a. *Echinococcus granulosus*
b. *Entamoeba histolytica*
c. *Schistosoma mansonii*
d. *Giardia lamblia*
e. *Clonorchis sinensis*

132) A 55-year-old homeless man presents with profuse haematemesis. He is unkempt and smells of alcohol. On examination his BP is 85/50 and pulse 130, and he has tender hepatomegaly and spider naevi. The most likely diagnosis is:

a. Oesophageal varices
b. Perforated peptic ulcer
c. Mallory–Weiss tear
d. Gastric varices
e. Angiodysplasia

133) Appropriate management after resuscitation includes all of the following EXCEPT:

a. Arrange urgent endoscopy
b. Crossmatch 6 units of blood
c. Consider Sengstaken–Blakemore tube to tamponade bleed
d. Administer octreotide
e. Commence cimetidine

134) You are obtaining consent from a patient for partial gastrectomy and discuss the risk of dumping syndrome. Which symptom is NOT associated with this syndrome?

a. Palpitations
b. Diarrhoea
c. Diaphoresis
d. Faintness
e. Nausea after eating

135) Causes of sclerosing cholangitis include all of the following EXCEPT:

a. Ulcerative colitis
b. Crohn's disease
c. Carcinoma
d. Gallstones
e. Previous biliary surgery

136) A 40-year-old woman undergoes laparoscopic cholecystectomy. This is converted to an open cholecystectomy on the table. Four days later she develops spiking temperatures to 40°C. Chest radiograph, MSU and blood cultures are clear. White cell count is raised with predominantly neutrophils. What is the next investigation?

a. CT scan of the abdomen
b. ERCP
c. Ultrasonography
d. Abdominal radiograph
e. Peritoneal tap

137) The most likely diagnosis is:

a. DVT
b. Pulmonary atelectasis
c. Subphrenic abscess
d. Retained stones in the common biliary duct
e. Anaphylaxis

138) A 70-year-old man undergoes right total knee replacement; 12 hours postoperatively you are called for poor urine output of 100 mL in the last 8 hours. On examination, he is pale and dyspnoeic. His BP is 88/58 with a pulse of 110. His pulse oximeter reads 98%. His preoperative Hb was 11 g/dL. He has been on fragmin preoperatively and postoperatively. You check the position of the Foley catheter. The next step is?

a. Take blood for urgent FBC and crossmatch
b. Insert a central line
c. Perform a 12-lead ECG
d. Arrange a ventilation–perfusion scan
e. Give boluses of intravenous fluids

139) Associations with gastric cancer include all of the following EXCEPT:

a. Pernicious anaemia
b. Atrophic gastritis
c. Blood group O
d. Acanthosis nigricans
e. Sister Mary Joseph's sign

140) A 50-year-old woman who is a secretary complains of tingling and numbness over the right thumb, index finger, middle finger and lateral half of the ring finger, worse at night. She also complains of weakness in holding a book. On examination there is weakness of the thumb abduction and wasting of the thenar muscles. The most likely diagnosis is:

a. Cervical spondylosis
b. Carpal tunnel syndrome
c. Multiple sclerosis
d. Rheumatoid arthritis
e. Myasthenia gravis

141) Treatment for carpal tunnel syndrome includes all of the following EXCEPT:

a. A splint
b. Diuretics
c. Depo-Medrone injection
d. Arthroscopic division of flexor retinaculum
e. Propranolol

142) A 65-year-old man presents with low back pain and urinary incontinence. On digital rectal examination (DRE), a hard nodular prostate is palpated. Appropriate investigations include all of the following EXCEPT:

    a. Prostate-specific antigen
    b. Isotope bone scan
    c. Transrectal biopsy
    d. Serum acid phosphatase
    e. Carcinoembryonic antigen

143) The carpal bone that is most likely to become necrotic following fracture is:

    a. Capitate
    b. Hamate
    c. Scaphoid
    d. Lunate
    e. Trapezoid

144) Risk factors for carcinoma of the oesophagus include all of the following EXCEPT:

    a. Alcohol
    b. Smoking
    c. Achalasia
    d. Barrett's oesophagus
    e. Blood group A

145) Clinical findings with pneumothorax include all of the following EXCEPT:

    a. Increased vocal fremitus
    b. Increased vocal resonance
    c. Raised percussion note
    d. Whispering pectoriloquy
    e. Tracheal shift to the same side

146) The following statements are true regarding blunt chest trauma EXCEPT:

    a. A contused lung goes into pulmonary oedema rapidly
    b. In a normal lung, bacteria are cleared in 4 hours
    c. In a contused lung, bacteria clear in 24 hours
    d. The first two ribs are the easiest to break
    e. Fractured ribs may be repaired by wire fixation

147) A 30-year-old woman presents with severe chest pain. She was a driver in a high-speed head-on collision. Her chest radiograph shows a widened mediastinum. The most likely diagnosis is:

   a. Haemothorax
   b. Pulmonary contusion
   c. Mediastinal mass
   d. Possible ruptured aorta
   e. Aortic aneurysm

148) Your next step would be:

   a. Arrange an urgent CT scan and then transfer the patient to a specialist centre
   b. Transfer the patient directly to a specialist centre
   c. Arrange urgent ultrasonography and then transfer the patient to a specialist centre
   d. Take the patient directly to theatre
   e. Treat the patient conservatively

149) The anatomy of the coronary arteries can be visualized by:

   a. Cardiac catheterization
   b. MUGA scan
   c. Positron emission tomography (PET) scan
   d. Thallium stress test
   e. Transoesophageal echocardiography

150) The following statements regarding undescended testes are correct EXCEPT:

   a. Undescended testes must be fixed by 1 year of age
   b. Ultrasonography is a useful investigation in children
   c. A CT scan is not indicated
   d. Most cases are retractile
   e. Surgery is offered to locate the testes via a high Jones' approach and then to fix the testes

151) The following statements regarding adenocarcinoma of the stomach are correct EXCEPT:

   a. The tumour is most commonly found in the fundus/cardia
   b. Intestinal gastric carcinoma has a better prognosis than diffuse type
   c. The investigation of choice is a double-contrast barium study + fibreoptic endoscopy
   d. Surgical laparotomy is the best method of staging this tumour
   e. Radical gastrectomy is offered for all stages of the tumour

152) A 50-year-old man presents with dysphagia. Endoscopy and biopsies reveal adenocarcinoma at the gastric fundus. CT scan confirms hepatic metastasis. The most appropriate treatment is:

    a. Radical gastrectomy
    b. Re-establish swallowing with recanalization with laser, intubation or bypass
    c. Chemotherapy with epirubicin, *cis*-platinum and continuous 5FU
    d. Radiotherapy
    e. Palliative resection

153) The treatment for established ARDS is:

    a. Intravenous broad-spectrum antibiotics
    b. Endotracheal intubation and intermittent positive-pressure ventilation
    c. Respiratory physiotherapy
    d. Fluid replacement with plasma expanders
    e. 100% oxygen by facemask

154) The following statements regarding management of burns are correct EXCEPT:

    a. Full-thickness burns are established by loss of sensation to pinprick
    b. Treatment should include intravenous broad-spectrum antibiotics
    c. Oral opiates are used for analgesia
    d. Fluid replacement is crucial
    e. Blood transfusion may be required

155) The most accurate investigation for diagnosing the site of a upper gastrointestinal bleed is:

    a. Double-contrast radiography
    b. Angiography
    c. Endoscopy
    d. Chest radiograph
    e. CT scan of the chest

156) Recognized methods of controlling an upper GI bleed include all of the following EXCEPT:

    a. Nd:YAG laser with endoscopy
    b. Endoscopic diathermy
    c. Endoscopic sclerotherapy
    d. Balloon tamponade
    e. Endoscopic intubation

157) Acute osteomyelitis is most commonly associated with:

a. *Streptococcus pneumoniae*
b. *Haemophilus influenzae*
c. Salmonellae
d. *Staphylococcus aureus*
e. *Streptococcus viridans*

158) A 50-year-old overweight banker complains of retrosternal chest pain, worse on lying flat and stooping down. He smokes 20 cigarettes a day. He takes no medication. The most likely diagnosis is:

a. Gastric ulcer
b. Angina
c. Duodenal ulcer
d. Costochondritis
e. Gastro-oesophageal reflux disease

159) What is the recommended treatment for *Helicobacter pylori* eradication?

a. Proton pump inhibitor + amoxicillin + metronidazole for 1 week
b. H$_2$-receptor blocker + amoxicillin + metronidazole for 2 weeks
c. Bismuth + amoxicillin + tetracycline for 6 weeks
d. Bismuth + clarithromycin + proton pump inhibitor for 2 weeks
e. Bismuth + amoxicillin + metronidazole for 2 weeks

160) Indications for surgery for duodenal ulcer include all of the following EXCEPT:

a. Pyloric stenosis
b. Perforation
c. Haemorrhage
d. Lack of patient compliance with medical treatment
e. Pain

161) Preoperative management of perforated duodenal ulcer includes all of the following EXCEPT:

a. Insert a nasogastric tube
b. Commence intravenous cefuroxime and metronidazole
c. Replete plasma volume with crystalloid
d. Insert a Foley catheter and maintain a urine output of 60 mL/h
e. Give diclofenac i.m. for analgesia

162) A 60-year-old man on intravenous cefuroxime and metronidazole for acute diverticulitis now presents with swinging pyrexia and a white cell count of 183×10^9/L. He is tender in the left iliac fossa but does not have peritoneal signs at this stage. The next step should be:

a. Obtain an urgent abdominal radiograph to exclude bowel obstruction
b. Obtain an upright chest radiograph to exclude perforation of a diverticulum
c. Request an ultrasound scan to exclude pericolic abscess
d. Expeditious surgery
e. Continue to treat conservatively with intravenous antibiotics

163) A 60-year-old man presents with vomiting and severe upper abdominal pain radiating to the back. He is sitting forward. He has a history of alcoholism. On examination temperature is 39°C, BP 90/50 and pulse 135/min. His abdomen is rigid with generalized tenderness. Pulse oximeter reads 80% O_2 saturation. Useful blood tests include all of the following EXCEPT:

a. FBC
b. Arterial blood gas
c. Serum amylase
d. Serum glucose
e. Clotting profile

164) Chest radiograph shows a small left-sided pleural effusion. Abdominal radiograph shows absent psoas shadow. Blood results are:

WBC	203×10^9/L
Hb	10 g/dL
Platelets	2503×10^9/L
Glucose	12 mmol/L
LDH	400 IU/L
AST	60 IU/L
γ-Glutamyltransferase	100 IU/L
Amylase	1200 IU/mL

The most likely diagnosis is:

a. Perforated peptic ulcer
b. Perforated gallbladder
c. Acute pancreatitis
d. Ruptured AAA (aortic abdominal aneurysm)
e. Alcoholic cirrhosis

165) A 50-year-old woman returns for her mammogram results. The mammogram reveals spiculation and finely scattered microcalcification. Fine-needle aspiration cytology (FNAC) confirms breast cancer. Further investigations for this patient include all of the following EXCEPT:

a. LFTs
b. Chest radiograph
c. A 12-lead ECG
d. Bone scan
e. Ultrasonography of the liver

166) A 20-year-old man attempts suicide by drinking sulphuric acid. Management should include all of the following EXCEPT:

a. Total parenteral nutrition
b. Gastrostomy
c. Nil by mouth
d. Steroids
e. Gentle dilatation with bougies after 3–4 weeks

167) Preoperative management for thyroidectomy should include:

a. ENT referral for vocal fold check
b. Type and crossmatch 2 units of blood
c. Serum calcium level
d. Subcutaneous fragmin
e. CT scan of the neck

168) Indications for thyroidectomy include all of the following EXCEPT:

a. Retrosternal goitre
b. Unsightly goitre
c. Solitary nodule
d. Fear of radiation
e. Myxoedema

169) A 25-year-old obese woman complains of difficulty breathing and swallowing. On examination her breathing is laboured and her trachea is displaced. You ask her to raise her arms above her head. She develops facial congestion and stridor. The most likely diagnosis is:

a. Retrosternal goitre
b. Tension pneumothorax
c. Cervical rib
d. Oesophageal carcinoma
e. Globus pharyngeus

170) The most appropriate initial investigation is:

   a. Plain chest radiograph + thoracic inlet view of the neck
   b. Ultrasonography of the neck
   c. Endoscopy
   d. Thyroid function tests
   e. Technetium scintiscan

171) A 70-year-old man presents with left lower abdominal pain and change in bowel habits. A barium enema shows a filling defect in the sigmoid colon. The most likely diagnosis is:

   a. Diverticulosis
   b. Carcinoma
   c. Crohn's disease
   d. Ulcerative colitis
   e. Familial adenomatous polyposis

172) Signs of venous hypertension include all of the following EXCEPT:

   a. Ankle flare
   b. Lipodermatosclerosis
   c. Varicose veins
   d. Cellulitis
   e. Shallow ulcers with sloping edges on the medial aspect of the leg

173) A 60-year-old man presents with acute right leg pain. On examination the leg is white, cold, desensate and pulseless. On-table angiography stops at the adductor canal. The next step is:

   a. Thrombolysis
   b. Reverse saphenous vein graft for femoral–popliteal bypass
   c. Primary stenting to the right iliac artery
   d. Dacron graft for femoral–popliteal bypass
   e. Reverse saphenous vein graft for femoral–posterior tibial bypass

174) A 50-year-old woman presents with pain and a cold right leg for 4 h. On examination her pulse is irregular with a rate of 120. She has a history of mitral valve disease. The most likely diagnosis is:

   a. Femoral artery embolism
   b. Popliteal aneurysm
   c. Femoral aneurysm
   d. Intermittent claudication
   e. Deep venous thrombosis

175) Appropriate investigations for Crohn's disease include all of the following EXCEPT:

   a. FBC
   b. Barium follow-through
   c. Colonoscopy
   d. ESR, CRP
   e. Sigmoidoscopy

176) A 50-year-old woman who underwent a thyroidectomy a week ago now presents with confusion. She also complains of perioral tingling. The most discriminating investigation is:

a. Serum glucose
b. LFTs
c. FBC and film
d. Thyroid function tests
e. Serum calcium

177) A 55-year-old man presents with a 2-day history of abdominal pain, flatulence and severe foul-smelling diarrhoea. He reports that he drank untreated water from a reservoir in the countryside. The most likely pathogen is:

a. Giardia
b. *E. coli*
c. *Leishmania donovania*
d. *Pityrosporum ovale*
e. *Plasmodium falciparum*

178) The patient was started on medications. He should be cautioned against drinking:

a. Lemonade
b. Grapefruit juice
c. Tea
d. Alcohol
e. Cranberry juice

179) A 30-year-old woman presents with drooping of the terminal phalanx of her middle right finger. She was making the bed at the time of injury. She is now unable to extend the tip of her finger. The most likely diagnosis is:

a. Bennett's fracture
b. Ulnar nerve injury
c. Median nerve injury
d. Mallet finger
e. Flexor digitorum profundus injury

180) A 40-year-old woman is scheduled for an elective laparoscopic cholecystectomy. Shortly after induction of general anaesthesia she develops a tachycardia, pyrexia and hypotension, and is clenching her jaw. The most likely diagnosis is:

a. Anaphylaxis
b. Suxamethonium apnoea
c. Malignant hyperthermia
d. Cardiac arrest
e. Respiratory arrest

181) The most likely causative agent is:

    a. Atropine
    b. Halogen
    c. Oxygen
    d. Suxamethonium
    e. Propofol

182) The intracellular substance that is markedly raised in this condition is:

    a. Calcium
    b. Potassium
    c. Hydrogen
    d. Nitrogen
    e. Sodium

183) A 30 year old who is a builder presents with a swelling in the upper arm that appears on elbow flexion. He says that he lifted a pile of bricks yesterday when he felt a snapping sensation in the upper arm region. The most likely diagnosis is:

    a. Adhesive capsulitis
    b. Rotator cuff injury
    c. Shoulder dislocation
    d. Rupture of long head of biceps
    e. Rupture of short head of biceps

184) A 60-year-old woman presents with postoperative oliguria. Urine output is 10 mL/h. The central venous pressure (CVP) line reads 10 mmHg. On lung auscultation there are râles present. The most appropriate management would be:

    a. Intravenous fluid bolus
    b. Furosemide
    c. Take blood for FBC
    d. Obtain a portable chest radiograph
    e. Commence intravenous broad-spectrum antibiotics

185) A 45-year-old man presents with right calf pain 1 week after a left hemicolectomy. On examination there is ankle oedema and positive Hoffman's sign. Ultrasound scan shows a clot in the right femoral vein. The most appropriate management is:

    a. Oral warfarin
    b. Intravenous heparin
    c. Oral aspirin
    d. Intravenous tPA (tissue plasminogen activator)
    e. Intravenous streptokinase

186) A 70-year-old man presents with episodes of weakness in the right arm which last for several minutes. He is a long-standing smoker. On examination he is hypertensive and on auscultation a loud left carotid bruit is heard. The most appropriate management is:

a. Carotid endarterectomy
b. Cerebral arteriography
c. Duplex ultrasonography of the carotid arteries
d. Initiation of heparin therapy
e. Transoesophageal echocardiography

187) General factors that delay healing include all of the following EXCEPT:

a. Thiamine deficiency
b. Vitamin C deficiency
c. Chemotherapy
d. Zinc deficiency
e. Uraemia

188) A 65-year-old woman presents with a 4-week history of progressive painless jaundice. Her urine is dark and stools pale. The most likely diagnosis is:

a. Cholecystitis
b. Pancreatic carcinoma
c. Hepatitis
d. Wilson's disease
e. Cirrhosis

189) A 55-year-old man presents to A&E after a night of drinking. He is unable to give a history as he is drunk but he complains of severe chest pain. On examination he is found to have surgical emphysema. The most likely diagnosis is:

a. Myocardial infarction
b. Pneumonia
c. Inhalation of foreign body
d. Ruptured oesophagus
e. Unstable angina

190) A 40-year-old man presents with a 1-month history of jaundice and malaise. His ferritin level is high and LFTs are elevated. The most likely diagnosis is:

a. Primary biliary cirrhosis
b. Pancreatic carcinoma
c. Haemochromatosis
d. Stomach carcinoma
e. Hepatitis

191) The most discriminating investigation is:

   a. ERCP
   b. Liver biopsy
   c. Liver ultrasonography
   d. Viral serology
   e. Serum mitochondrial antibodies

192) A positive Froment's sign can be elicited in:

   a. Median nerve lesion
   b. Ulnar nerve lesion
   c. Axillary nerve lesion
   d. Radial nerve lesion
   e. Accessory nerve lesion

193) Repair of an abdominal aortic aneurysm is advocated when the size of the aneurysm is:

   a. >7 cm
   b. >6.5 cm
   c. >5.5 cm
   d. <4 cm
   e. <5.5 cm

194) A 20-year-old presents with a swollen, tender finger. A radiograph shows a transverse, undisplaced fracture of the proximal phalanx. The most appropriate treatment is:

   a. Closed reduction and cast immobilization
   b. Open reduction and plating
   c. Buddy strapping
   d. Sling
   e. Open reduction and Kirschner wire fixation

195) An 80-year-old woman presents to A&E after a fall directly on to her hip; she is now unable to weight bear. The leg is shorter and externally rotated. She cannot lift her leg. The most likely diagnosis is:

   a. Femoral shaft fracture
   b. Fractured patella
   c. Pelvic fracture
   d. Fractured tibial spine
   e. Intertrochanteric fracture

2. Surgery: EMQ Questions

Theme: diagnosis of abdominal pain

Options

A. Acute appendicitis
B. Diverticular disease
C. Abdominal aortic aneurysm
D. Perforated peptic ulcer
E. Crohn's disease
F. Ulcerative colitis
G. Acute pancreatitis
H. Chronic active hepatitis
I. Acute viral hepatitis
J. Pseudo-obstruction
K. Acute cholecystitis
L. Acute diverticulitis

For each presentation below, choose the SINGLE most likely diagnosis from the list of options. Each option may be used once, more than once or not at all.

1) A 20-year-old man presents with colicky periumbilical pain which shifts to the RIF, fever and loss of appetite.

2) A 48-year-old man presents with severe epigastric pain radiating to the back. He is noted to have some bruising in the flanks.

3) A 42-year-old woman presents with anorexia, abdominal pain and increasing jaundice. She is asthmatic and takes methyldopa for hypertension.

4) A 50-year-old man presents with sudden left-sided iliac fossa pain and a mild pyrexia. He complains of long-standing constipation. There is no weight loss. Full blood count shows a leucocytosis.

5) A 78-year-old woman with stable angina presents with massive abdominal distension 10 days after a total hip replacement.

Theme: diagnosis of breast diseases

Options

A. Fibroadenoma
B. Fibrocystic disease
C. Galactocele
D. Intraductal papilloma
E. Mammary duct ectasia
F. Breast cancer
G. Cystosarcoma phylloides
H. Breast abscess
I. Fat necrosis
J. Paget's disease
K. Eczema of the nipple

For each patient below, choose the SINGLE most likely diagnosis from the list of options. Each option may be used once, more than once or not at all.

6) A 28-year-old woman presents with a solitary 3-cm freely mobile painless nodule. She also complains of a serous nipple discharge and axillary lymphadenopathy.

7) A 36-year-old woman presents with multiple and bilateral cystic breast swellings which are noted to be particularly painful and tender premenstrually. She states that during pregnancy the symptoms improved.

8) A 50-year-old woman presents with nipple discharge, nipple retraction, dilatation of ducts, and chronic intraductal and periductal inflammation. The diagnosis is confirmed by breast biopsy and no further treatment is required.

9) A 50-year-old woman presents with an eczematous appearance to her nipple and areola. It is associated with a discrete nodule that is attached to the overlying skin.

10) A 33-year-old lactating woman presents with a 1-week history of a painful, erythematous breast lump and pyrexia. She has tried a course of antibiotics to no avail.

Theme: causes of neck lumps

Options

A. Branchial cyst
B. Ludwig's angina
C. Parotitis
D. Thyroglossal cyst
E. Dermoid cyst
F. Parapharyngeal abscess
G. Thyroid swelling
H. Sialectasis
I. Laryngocele
J. Pharyngeal pouch
K. Reactive lymphadenitis

For each presentation below, choose the SINGLE most likely cause from the list of options. Each option may be used once, more than once or not at all.

11) A 45-year-old clarinet player presents with a neck swelling that expands with forced expiration.

12) A 4-year-old boy presents with a small midline neck swelling which moves on swallowing. It is painless, mobile, transilluminates and fluctuates.

13) A 26-year-old man, after a trip to the dentist for a toothache, presents with a tender neck swelling, pyrexia and pain on swallowing. The tonsils are not inflamed.

14) A 30-year-old man presents with a 5-cm neck swelling anterior to the sternomastoid muscle on the left side in its upper third. He states that the swelling has been treated with antibiotics for infection in the past.

15) A 20-year-old man presents with a painful swelling under his jaw. On examination he has trismus and is dribbling saliva.

Theme: treatment of postoperative pain

Options

A. Aspirin tablets
B. Diclofenac suppositories
C. Tramadol tablets
D. Patient-controlled analgesia (PCA) with morphine
E. Intercostal nerve blocks
F. Epidural analgesia
G. Carbamazepine
H. Paracetamol tablets
I. Diamorphine
J. Intramuscular pethidine

For each case below, choose the SINGLE most appropriate treatment from the list of options. Each option may be used once, more than once or not at all.

16) A 33-year-old man requires analgesia following an exploratory laparotomy and splenectomy.

17) A 55-year-old woman with terminal metastatic breast carcinoma requires long-term analgesia following a radical mastectomy.

18) A 40-year-old man complains of phantom limb pain following a below-the-knee amputation.

19) A 25-year-old man underwent excision of a sebaceous cyst under local anaesthesia. He uses a salbutamol inhaler on a regular basis.

20) A 60-year-old man requires analgesia following a total thyroidectomy.

Theme: investigation of postoperative complications

Options

A. Chest radiograph
B. Serum calcium
C. A 12-lead ECG
D. Ultrasonography of the abdomen
E. Serum glucose
F. Midstream specimen of urine
G. Thyroid function tests
H. Pulmonary angiogram
I. Bladder ultrasonography
J. Serum haemoglobin

For each presentation below, choose the SINGLE most confirmatory investigation from the list of options. Each option may be used once, more than once or not at all.

21) A 55-year-old man post-thyroidectomy presents with tetany. On tapping the preauricular region, the facial muscles begin to twitch.

22) A 50-year-old man after coronary artery bypass graft surgery presents with fever and severe epigastric pain.

23) A 70-year-old woman after a dynamic hip screw for a right neck of femur fracture presents with pallor, tachycardia and hypotension. Oxygen saturation is 90%. The rest of her examination is normal.

24) A 65-year-old man, 10 days after right total hip replacement, presents with sudden breathlessness and collapses. On examination he is noted to have a pleural rub, increased JVP and a swollen right leg.

25) A 35-year-old woman who is a primigravida complains of inability to void after a caesarean section. She denies dysuria but complains of fullness. She was treated with an epidural for analgesia.

Theme: investigation of abdominal pain

Options

A. Ultrasonography of the abdomen
B. Rectal examination
C. Upper GI endoscopy
D. Barium meal
E. Sigmoidoscopy
F. Colonoscopy
G. CT scan of the abdomen
H. Kidneys, ureters and bladder (KUB) radiograph
I. Pelvic ultrasonography
J. Laparoscopy
K. Erect chest radiograph

For each presentation below, choose the SINGLE most discriminating investigation from the list of options. Each option may be used once, more than once or not at all.

26) A 60-year-old man complains of severe colicky pain from his right flank radiating to his groin. Urinalysis reveals trace blood cells.

27) A 25-year-old woman complains of severe lower abdominal pain and increasing abdominal girth. Urine hCG is negative.

28) A 60-year-old obese man complains of severe epigastric pain radiating to his back. The pain is relieved by eating and is worse at night.

29) A 65-year-old hypertensive man presents with lower abdominal pain and back pain. An expansive abdominal mass is palpated lateral and superior to the umbilicus.

30) An 80-year-old woman with rheumatoid arthritis presents with severe epigastric pain and vomiting. She also complains of shoulder tip pain.

Theme: diagnosis of hearing problems

Options

A. Presbyacusis
B. Cerumen
C. Acute suppurative otitis media
D. Otitis externa
E. Chronic secretory otitis media
F. Barotrauma
G. Chronic suppurative otitis media
H. Dead ear
I. Otosclerosis
J. Temporal bone fracture
K. Osteogenesis imperfecta

For each patient below, choose the SINGLE most likely diagnosis from the list of options. Each option may be used once, more than once or not at all.

31) A 70-year-old man presents with gradual deterioration of hearing in both ears. The Weber tuning fork test is non-lateralizing and the Rinne test is positive on both sides. The tympanic membranes are intact and healthy.

32) A 60-year-old man presents with unilateral earache, diminished hearing and foul-smelling discharge. The external auditory meatus is oedematous and the canal is stenosed. The discharge is white and creamy in nature.

33) A 40-year-old woman presents with diminished hearing in the right ear. She denies earache or discharge. She is noted to have blue sclerae. The tympanic membrane is normal. The Weber tuning fork test lateralizes to the right side and the Rinne test is negative on the right.

34) A 4-year-old girl presents to her GP with diminished hearing noted by the school. On examination there is a bulging yellow tympanic membrane on the right alone.

35) A 70-year-old woman presents with longstanding deafness in the left ear. The Weber test lateralizes to the right and the Rinne test is negative on the left.

Theme: diagnosis of conditions of the hand

Options

A. Volkmann's ischaemic contracture
B. Dupuytren's contracture
C. Carpal tunnel syndrome
D. Claw hand
E. Raynaud's phenomenon
F. Scleroderma
G. Rheumatoid arthritis
H. Paronychia
I. Psoriasis
J. Koilonychia
K. Glomus tumour
L. Subungual haematoma

For each presentation below, choose the SINGLE most likely diagnosis from the list of options. Each option may be used once, more than once or not at all.

36) A 20-year-old woman presents with a painful fingertip that throbs and has kept the patient up all night. The skin at the base and side of the nail is red, tender and bulging.

37) A 30-year-old woman presents with a painful fingernail. On examination there is a small purple–red spot beneath the nail. She denies trauma to the finger.

38) A 60-year-old man with acromegaly presents with pins and needles in the index and middle fingers of his right hand, worse at night.

39) A 20-year-old man presents with fingers that are permanently flexed in his right hand. However, the deformity is abolished by flexion of the wrist. He admits to trauma to his elbow recently. He also complains of pins and needles.

40) A 20-year-old woman complains of intermittent pain in her fingertips. She describes the fingers undergoing colour changes from white to blue and then to red. The symptoms are worse in the winter.

Theme: causes of haematemesis

Options

A. Chronic peptic ulceration
B. Gastritis
C. Oesophageal varices
D. Mallory–Weiss tear
E. Carcinoma of the oesophagus
F. Carcinoma of the stomach
G. Oesophagitis
H. Haemophilia
I. Epistaxis
J. Angiodysplasia
K. Peutz–Jeghers syndrome
L. Ehlers–Danlos syndrome

For each case below, choose the SINGLE most likely cause from the list of options. Each option may be used once, more than once or not at all.

41) A 17-year-old girl presents with haematemesis after several episodes of vomiting. Her mother informs you that she is 'very body conscious'.

42) A 50-year-old man presents with massive haematemesis. He is noted to have freckles on his lower lips.

43) A 60-year-old man with alcohol dependence presents with massive haematemesis and shock. He is noted to have finger clubbing and ascites.

44) A 70-year-old man with chronic hoarseness presents with retrosternal chest pain and haematemesis. He has a history of achalasia and has lost 1 stone in weight.

45) A 65-year-old man presents with haematemesis. He is noted to have an enlarged left supraclavicular node, ascites and anaemia.

Theme: causes of abdominal masses

Options

A. Psoas abscess
B. Appendicitis
C. Tuberculosis
D. Crohn's disease
E. Diverticulitis
F. Carcinoma in the sigmoid colon
G. Carcinoma of the caecum
H. Obstruction of the common bile duct by a calculus
I. Carcinoma of the pancreas
J. Ovarian cyst
K. Mesenteric cyst

For each case below, choose the SINGLE most likely cause from the list of options. Each option may be used once, more than once or not at all.

46) A 40-year-old man presents with fever, painless jaundice and a palpable gallbladder.

47) A 30-year-old woman presents with colicky abdominal pain and distension. On examination a smooth, mobile, spherical mass is palpated in the centre of her abdomen. A fluid thrill is elicited and the mass is dull to percussion.

48) A 20-year-old man presents with fever, abdominal and back pain, and a mass in the right iliac fossa. The swelling is soft, tender, dull and compressible. It extends below the groin. He denies nausea, vomiting or diarrhoea.

49) A 50-year-old man presents with a dull ache in the right iliac fossa and diarrhoea. A freely mobile mass is palpated in the right iliac fossa. The rectum is normal and the faeces contain blood.

50) A 55-year-old man presents with severe left iliac fossa pain, nausea and chronic constipation. A tender, sausage-shaped mass is palpated in the left iliac fossa.

Theme: causes of shock

Options

A. Pulmonary embolism
B. Myocardial ischaemia
C. Cardiac tamponade
D. Trauma
E. Burns
F. Sepsis
G. Anaphylaxis
H. Major surgery
I. Ruptured aortic aneurysm
J. Ectopic pregnancy
K. Addisonian crisis
L. Hypothyroidism
M. Acute pancreatitis

For each patient below, choose the SINGLE most likely cause from the list of options. Each option may be used once, more than once or not at all.

51) A 50-year-old man arrives at A&E in shock. His BP is 80/50. The heart sounds are muffled. The JVP increases with inspiration.

52) A 30-year-old woman presents to A&E in respiratory distress and shock. She is noted to have stridor. Her lips are swollen and blue.

53) A 55-year-old man presents to A&E with severe abdominal pain, vomiting and shock. The pain is in the upper abdomen and radiates to the back. He takes diuretics. The abdomen is rigid, and the radiograph shows absent psoas shadow.

54) A 60-year-old woman presents to A&E in shock with continuous abdominal pain radiating to her back. The abdomen is rigid with an expansile abdominal mass.

55) A 35-year-old woman presents to A&E in shock with a BP of 80/50 and tachycardia. She is confused and weak. Her husband states that she forgot to take her prednisolone tablets with her on holiday and has missed several doses.

Theme: treatment of fractures and dislocations

Options

A. Kocher's method
B. AO cannulated screws
C. Bedrest
D. Open reduction and a Kirschner wire
E. Buddy strapping
F. Reconstructive surgery with internal graft or implant augmentation
G. Physiotherapy for strengthening exercises
H. Austin Moore hemiarthroplasty
I. Dynamic hip screw
J. Total hip replacement
K. Open reduction and internal fixation

For each of the cases below, choose the SINGLE most appropriate treatment from the list of options. Each option may be used once, more than once or not at all.

56) A 50-year-old fit man presents with a right hip fracture. On radiograph the fracture line is subcapital.

57) A 20-year-old man who is an athlete twists his knee on holiday while skiing. On examination he has a positive drawer sign with the tibia sliding anteriorly.

58) A 70-year-old woman presents with a left hip fracture. On a radiograph the fracture line is intertrochanteric.

59) A 40-year-old woman sprains her wrist. She complains of persistent pain and tenderness over the dorsum distal to Lister's tubercle. Radiographs show a large gap between the scaphoid and the lunate. In the lateral view, the lunate is tilted dorsally and the scaphoid anteriorly.

60) A 30-year-old man who is a basketball player presents with severe pain in his shoulder. He is holding his arm with the opposite hand. He explains that he fell on an outstretched hand. The radiograph shows overlapping shadows of the humeral head and glenoid fossa, with the head lying below and medial to the socket. There is also a fracture of the neck of the humerus.

Theme: management of traumatic injuries

Options

A. Peritoneal lavage
B. Observation and angiography
C. Closed thoracotomy tube drainage
D. Pressure dressing
E. Cricothyroidotomy
F. Nasogastric tube suction and observation
G. Surgical repair of the flexor digitorum superficialis tendon
H. Surgical repair of the flexor digitorum profundus tendon
I. Urgent surgical exploration
J. Debridement and repair
K. Endotracheal intubation
L. Needle pericardiocentesis
M. Fasciotomy

For each case below, choose the SINGLE most appropriate management from the list of options. Each option may be used once, more than once or not at all.

61) A 23-year-old man presents to A&E having been stabbed in the neck. He complains of difficulty swallowing and talking. He has no stridor. On examination there is a small penetrating wound with diffuse neck swelling.

62) A 12-year-old boy presents with a hand injury sustained while attempting to catch a ball. On examination he is unable to bend the tip of his right middle finger.

63) A 35-year-old woman is brought into A&E acutely short of breath. Respiratory rate is 50/min. She was involved in a road traffic accident. There are no breath sounds auscultated on the left. The trachea is deviated to the right.

64) An 18-year-old man sustains a stab wound to the right thigh. On examination there is a large haematoma over the thigh and weak distal pulses. He is unable to move his foot and complains of pins and needles in his foot.

65) A 30-year-old woman involved in a head-on car collision presents with diffuse abdominal pain. An upright chest radiograph shows elevation of the diaphragm with a stomach gas bubble in the left lower lung field.

Theme: diagnosis of gastrointestinal conditions

Options

A. Hepatoma
B. Oesophageal varices
C. Mallory–Weiss tear
D. Perforated peptic ulcer
E. Fractured rib
F. Haematoma of the rectus sheath
G. Umbilical hernia
H. Sigmoid volvulus
I. Splenic rupture
J. Pancreatic pseudocyst
K. Divarication of rectus abdominis
L. Acute pancreatitis

For each case below, choose the SINGLE most likely diagnosis from the list of options. Each option may be used once, more than once or not at all.

66) A 50-year-old man with alcohol problems presents with nausea, vomiting and epigastric pain. On examination there is a palpable epigastric mass. The amylase is raised. A CT scan of the abdomen shows a round well-circumscribed mass in the epigastrium.

67) A 40-year-old multiparous woman presents with a midline abdominal mass. The mass is non-tender and appears when she is straining. On examination the midline mass is visible when she raises her head off the examining bed.

68) A 19-year-old man presents with sudden severe upper abdominal pain after being tackled during rugby practice. He was recently diagnosed with glandular fever.

69) A 7-year-old girl presents with a spontaneous massive haematemesis.

70) A 55-year-old man with alcohol problems presents with vomiting 800 mL blood. Blood pressure is 80/50 with a pulse rate of 120. Ascites is noted.

Theme: management of postoperative complications

Options

A. Intravenous dantrolene sodium
B. Intravenous calcium gluconate
C. Blood transfusion
D. Blood cultures
E. Obtain chest radiograph
F. Midstream urine collection for culture
G. Intravenous broad-spectrum antibiotics
H. Insulin in dextrose
I. Foley catheterization
J. Obtain abdominal radiograph
K. Check full blood count

For each case below, choose the SINGLE most appropriate management option from the list of options. Each option may be used once, more than once or not at all.

71) A 30-year-old woman post-appendectomy develops high fever of 42°C, hypotension and mottled cyanosis in the recovery room. She received halothane inhalational gas in surgery. She was noted to have trismus during intubation.

72) A 40-year-old man complains of circumoral numbness following thyroidectomy. Tapping over his preauricular region elicits facial twitching.

73) A 50-year-old man post-nephrectomy becomes febrile, confused, tachypnoeic and tachycardic. He was recently advanced to a soft diet. There are no bowel sounds.

74) A 60-year-old man complains of lower abdominal pain post-cholecystectomy. On examination the bladder is palpable at the umbilicus.

75) A 70-year-old woman becomes tachypnoeic after total hip replacement. She is pale and hypotensive.

Theme: diagnosis of chest injuries

Options

A. Flail chest
B. Tension pneumothorax
C. Haemothorax
D. Cardiac tamponade
E. Rib fracture
F. Pulmonary contusion
G. Myocardial contusion
H. Diaphragmatic rupture
I. Open pneumothorax

For each case below, choose the SINGLE most likely diagnosis from the list of options. Each option may be used once, more than once or not at all.

76) A 50-year-old man sustains blunt trauma to his chest and presents with marked dyspnoea. A nasogastric tube is inserted to decompress his stomach. On chest radiograph the nasogastric tube is seen in the left side of the chest.

77) A 55-year-old man involved in a road traffic accident complains of chest pain. He was driving the car and rear-ended the front car with some force. A friction rub is elicited. ECG shows multiple premature ventricular ectopic beats.

78) A 30-year-old man is stabbed in the back and is brought to A&E in respiratory distress. Blood pressure is 90/50 with a pulse rate of 110. There are dull breath sounds over his left chest. You leave the knife *in situ*.

79) A 40-year-old man is stabbed in the chest and is brought to A&E with shortness of breath. A 4-cm stab wound is noted and the wound is heard to 'suck' with each breath.

80) A 30-year-old man is stabbed in the left side of his chest and is brought to A&E. He is short of breath and restless. The chest is clear to auscultation. There is a rise in venous pressure with inspiration. Chest radiograph shows a globular shaped heart.

Theme: management of head injuries

Options

A. Admit for neurological observation
B. Assess adequacy of breathing
C. Removal of penetrating object
D. Discharge with head injury advice
E. Detailed neurological assessment
F. Airway assessment with cervical spine control
G. Assess circulation and maintain adequate perfusion
H. Neurosurgical consultation
I. Obtain urgent CT scan of the head
J. Intubate the patient
K. Pronounce the patient as deceased

For each case below, choose the SINGLE most appropriate form of management from the list of options. Each option may be used once, more than once or not at all.

81) A 30-year-old cyclist is struck by a car in a head-on collision and arrives intubated to A&E. on arrival his Glasgow Coma Scale score is 3. The pupils are fixed and dilated.

82) A 60-year-old man is brought to A&E following assault and battery to the head. He has a facemask and reservoir bag delivering 15 L/min of oxygen and a stiff cervical collar, and is attached to an intravenous drip. He has no spontaneous eye opening except to pain, makes incomprehensible sounds and does not obey commands. He demonstrates flexion withdrawal to painful stimuli. On suction he has no gag reflex.

83) A 20-year-old man involved in an RTA presents to A&E with a large open scalp wound, multiple facial injuries and a deformed right tibia.

84) A 40-year-old man is brought to A&E with a knife impaled in his occiput.

85) A 30-year-old woman involved in a RTA with multiple injuries is brought to A&E intubated with adequate oxygen delivery. Blood pressure is 80/50 with a pulse of 120.

Theme: management of back pain

Options

A. Obtain chest radiograph
B. Bedrest for 2 weeks
C. Rest for 2 days with analgesia
D. Physiotherapy
E. Urinalysis
F. Investigate for underlying tumour or other bone pathology
G. Urgent orthopaedic referral for surgical decompression
H. Routine orthopaedic referral for decompression of nerve root
I. Abdominal ultrasonography

For each case below, choose the SINGLE most appropriate management option from the list of options. Each option may be used once, more than once or not at all.

86) A 40-year-old man complains of lower back pain after moving heavy furniture. He has no associated nerve root findings.

87) A 50-year-old woman complains of back pain worse at night. A radiograph of her spine shows crush fractures of two vertebrae. She denies trauma.

88) A 60-year-old man presents with back pain radiating bilaterally below the knees. On examination he has saddle anaesthesia, urinary incontinence and loss of anal tone.

89) A 50-year-old woman complains of chronic lower back pain radiating into her buttocks. There is no evidence of nerve root entrapment.

90) A 30-year-old man complains of back pain radiating below the knee. On examination he has sensory loss over the lateral aspect of the right calf and medial aspect of the right foot. He is unable to dorsiflex his great toe. He has tried bedrest for 6 weeks!

Theme: diagnosis of head injuries

Options

A. Basal skull fracture
B. Depressed skull fracture
C. Compound skull fracture
D. Diffuse axonal injury
E. Concussion
F. Subdural haematoma
G. Intracerebral haemorrhage
H. Extradural haematoma
I. Open skull fracture
J. Brain contusion

For each case below, choose the SINGLE most likely diagnosis from the list of options. Each option may be used once, more than once or not at all.

91) A 30-year-old woman involved in an RTA is brought by ambulance to A&E. There is bruising of the mastoid process and periorbital haematoma. On otoscopic examination there is bleeding behind the tympanic membrane.

92) A 60-year-old man was kicked in the head a week ago. He is brought to A&E in an unconscious state. He smells of alcohol. On examination he has a rising BP and unequal pupils. His GCS is 8.

93) A 40-year-old man was struck in the head by a cricket ball. He had an episode of loss of consciousness lasting 5 min. The patient now complains of headache. He has no lateralizing signs on neurological examination.

94) A 50-year-old man with a history of epilepsy has a fit and strikes the side of his head on the edge of the bathtub. He is dazed and complains of headache. Skull radiograph reveals a linear fracture of the parietal area. His level of consciousness diminishes.

95) A 60-year-old man is struck in the head with a dustbin lid and presents with an open scalp wound. Skull radiograph confirms an underlying skull fracture. The dura is intact.

Theme: treatment of shoulder region injuries

Options

A. Broad arm sling
B. Collar and cuff sling
C. Rest and analgesia, then mobilize
D. Injection of local anaesthetic and steroids
E. Manipulation under anaesthesia
F. Traction on the arm in 90° of abduction and externally rotate the arm
G. Hippocratic technique
H. Kocher's technique
I. Surgical repair

For each case below, choose the SINGLE most appropriate treatment from the list of options. Each option may be used once, more than once or not at all.

96) A 20-year-old man presents with shoulder pain and decreased range of movement after being struck in the upper back. A radiograph reveals fracture of the scapula.

97) A 60-year-old man presents with pain in the upper arm. On examination there is a low bulge of the muscle belly of the long head of biceps.

98) A 50-year-old man complains of pain in his shoulder. The pain is elicited in abduction between an arc of 60° and one of 120°. He reports that he has always had shoulder trouble.

99) A 20-year-old man who is a rugby player falls on to the point of his shoulder and complains of shoulder tip pain. The lateral end of the clavicle is very prominent.

100) A 30-year-old man who has been hiking falls onto his outstretched hand and injures his right shoulder. On examination there is loss of the rounded shoulder contour with prominence of the acromion. On palpation there is a gap beneath the acromion and the humeral head is palpable in the axilla. The nearest hospital is 6 hours' hike away, and you are alone with him up on the mountain. You cannot obtain a signal on your mobile phone. You decide to treat the patient.

Theme: causes of a painful foot

Options

A. Morton's neuroma
B. Stress fracture
C. Avulsion fracture
D. Jones's fracture
E. Hallux fracture
F. Plantar fasciitis
G. Osteochondritis – Freiberg's disease
H. Metatarsalgia
I. Osteochondritis – Kohler's disease
J. Bunion
K. Gout

For each case below, choose the SINGLE most likely cause from the list of options. Each option may be used once, more than once or not at all.

101) A 50-year-old man presents with pain over the medial calcaneum and pain on dorsiflexion and eversion of the forefoot.

102) A 60-year-old man complains of continual pain in his forefoot worse when walking. A radiograph shows widening and flattening of the second metatarsal head and degenerative changes in the metatarsophalangeal joint.

103) A 50-year-old woman complains of shooting pains in her right foot when walking. There is tenderness in the third/fourth toe interspace.

104) A 30-year-old soldier complains of pain in his foot when weight bearing. A radiograph shows no fracture. There is tenderness around the proximal fifth metatarsal bone.

105) A 20-year-old man complains of pain over the lateral aspect of his right foot. A radiograph shows a transverse fracture of the basal shaft of the fifth metatarsal bone.

Theme: management of ENT emergencies

Options

A. Give nifedipine 10 mg
B. Obtain a barium swallow
C. Obtain a sialogram
D. Advise patient to drink more fluids and avoid citrus fruits
E. List for bronchoscopy
F. List for rigid oesophagoscopy
G. Intramuscular Buscopan
H. Insert two large-bore intravenous cannulas and run Gelofusine
I. Ligate sphenopalatine artery in theatre
J. Consult a haematologist
K. Check INR

For each patient below, choose the SINGLE most appropriate management option from the list of options. Each option may be used once, more than once or not at all.

106) A 70-year-old woman presents with severe epistaxis. Her BP is 205/115. She has no prior history of hypertension. She denies aspirin or warfarin use. Bloods are taken and an intravenous line is inserted. She continues to bleed profusely through her nose packs.

107) A 60-year-old man on warfarin 6 mg once daily for a previous DVT now presents with right-sided epistaxis. BP is 120/70 with a pulse rate of 90. He has no visible vessels in Little's area. He continues to bleed through the nose pack.

108) A 60-year-old woman presents with a piece of chicken stuck in her throat. Soft-tissue neck radiograph reveals a calcified bolus at the level of the cricopharyngeus.

109) A 70-year-old woman complains of mashed potato stuck in her throat since dinner. She is not distressed. She is able to sip water.

110) A 30-year-old man complains of intermittent unilateral cheek swelling with eating. On examination no swelling is palpated, and the oral cavity is clear.

Theme: investigations of surgical disease

Options

A. Gastrografin swallow
B. Upright chest radiograph
C. Abdominal radiograph
D. Full blood count
E. Mesenteric arteriogram
F. CT scan of the abdomen
G. Technetium-99m radioactive scan
H. Abdominal ultrasonography
I. Serum urea and electrolytes
J. Stool culture

For each case below, choose the SINGLE most discriminating investigation from the list of options. Each option may be used once, more than once or not at all.

111) A 60-year-old man, postoperative to rigid oesophagoscopy and removal of a foreign body, now presents with substernal pain, fever and tachypnoea.

112) A 65-year-old man with a history of cirrhosis presents with massive rectal bleeding and right lower quadrant pain. Nasogastric tube lavage reveals no blood in the stomach. Colonoscopy reveals no varices. You suspect angiodysplasia of the caecum.

113) A 20-year-old man presents with passage of frank blood and clots from his rectum. Blood tests, barium enema and upper GI series are all normal.

114) A 60-year-old man with lung cancer has elevated liver function tests. You suspect metastatic disease.

115) A 65-year-old man with alcohol problems now presents with a tender palpable midline mass. He was recently hospitalized for acute pancreatitis 2 weeks. The serum amylase is raised. You now suspect that he has a pancreatic pseudocyst.

Theme: treatment of abdominal pain

Options

A. ERCP and endoscopic sphincterotomy
B. Laparoscopic cholecystectomy
C. Intravenous fluids, intravenous antibiotics and analgesia
D. Subtotal colectomy, mucus fistula and permanent ileostomy
E. Laparotomy
F. Mesalazine
G. Panproctocolectomy
H. Hartmann's procedure

For each case below, choose the SINGLE most appropriate treatment from the list of options. Each option may be used once, more than once or not at all.

116) A 20-year-old woman presents with recurrent bloody diarrhoea and crampy abdominal pain. Sigmoidoscopy and biopsy confirm ulcerative colitis.

117) A 25-year-old man involved in an RTA sustains blunt trauma to his upper abdomen. He complains of left shoulder pain and diffuse abdominal pain. He becomes increasingly tachycardic and hypotensive and develops peritoneal signs.

118) A 40-year-old woman presents with pyrexia and right upper quadrant abdominal pain. The white cell count is 14 with elevated neutrophils. Both the chest radiograph and the abdominal radiograph are unremarkable.

119) A 50-year-old man presents with fever, right upper quadrant pain and jaundice. Ultrasonography reveals a dilated common bile duct.

120) A 30-year-old man presents with severe, intractable abdominal pain. He is pyrexial, tachycardic and has marked abdominal distension. On radiograph the colon is noted to have a transverse diameter of 7 cm.

Theme: rectal pain

Options

A. Fissure *in ano*
B. Fistula *in ano*
C. Haemorrhoids
D. Proctalgia fugax
E. Perianal haematoma
F. Carcinoma of the rectum
G. Crohn's disease
H. Ulcerative colitis
I. Ischaemic colitis
J. Diverticulitis

For each case below, choose the SINGLE most likely diagnosis from the list of options. Each option may be used once, more than once or not at all.

121) A 25-year-old woman presents with a history of intermittent rectal pain. She describes the episodes as a sudden severe shooting-like pain. Examination and sigmoidoscopy are normal.

122) A 50-year-old man presents with a 2-month history of worsening diarrhoea and bleeding per rectum. On sigmoidoscopy there is a 2-cm ulcer found at 10 cm in the anal canal.

123) A 25-year-old woman comes to you with pain on defecation with occasional blood on the toilet paper. Rectal examination is discontinued due to severe pain.

124) A 31-year-old woman complains of a 2-month history of intense pain on defecation. She reports that this started after the birth of her first child. On examination a pink-/purple-coloured mass at the anus is seen and is mildly tender on palpation.

125) A 35-year-old man is found to have an ulcer on colonoscopy. He is also noted to have a fissure *in ano* and a number of perianal skin tags

Theme: breast cancer

Options

A. Pathological fracture
B. Cerebral metastases
C. Hypocalcaemia
D. Hypercalcaemia
E. Lymphoedema
F. Spinal cord compression
G. Pleural effusion
H. Liver metastasis
I. Peritoneal recurrence
J. Local recurrence
K. Diabetes mellitus
L. Lymphangitis carcinomatosis

For each case below, choose the SINGLE most likely diagnosis from the list of options. Each option may be used once, more than once or not at all.

126) A 45-year-old woman who was diagnosed with breast cancer 3 years ago presents with breathlessness. She has had a left mastectomy and lymph node clearance. On examination breath sounds on the left are reduced and there is dullness to percussion.

127) A 35-year-old woman treated 1 year ago for breast cancer presents with a 2-day history of confusion. She is drowsy and disoriented. Her husband reports that she had been complaining of severe thirst for the past week.

128) A 45-year old woman who was treated 3 years ago for breast cancer now presents with back pain and numbness of the legs. She has been constipated for the last 24 hours.

129) A 43-year-old woman who was treated 2 years ago for breast cancer presents with confusion, headache and vomiting. On examination she is drowsy but has no focal neurological sings. On examination, papilloedema is present.

130) A 40-year-old woman has been diagnosed with metastatic cancer. She presents to A&E after a fall and is complaining of thigh pain.

Theme: traumatic injuries

Options

A. Bladder rupture
B. Renal contusion
C. Oesophageal injury
D. Pancreatic injury
E. Aortic rupture
F. Liver laceration
G. Renal pelvis avulsion
H. Splenic rupture
I. Diaphragmatic rupture
J. Stomach injury

For each case below, choose the SINGLE most likely diagnosis from the list of options. Each option may be used once, more than once or not at all.

131) A 35-year-old man is involved in a fight. He receives hard blows to the upper abdomen. On examination there is bruising in the left upper abdomen. Although he was initially stable he now develops a tachycardia and hypotension.

132) A 40-year-old woman is involved in an RTA. She was the driver of the car but was not wearing a seatbelt. She complains of chest pain. A chest radiograph reveals obliteration of the aortic knob.

133) A 30-year-old man is involved in an RTA. He is breathless and complains of chest and shoulder pain. On examination breath sounds are reduced on the left side. A chest radiograph shows a high left hemidiaphragm.

134) A 25-year-old woman jumps out of a third storey window and lands on her right side. She complains of right flank tenderness. A radiograph reveals fractures of the eleventh and twelfth ribs. A CT contrast scan is normal.

135) A 20-year-old man is stabbed in the upper abdomen. He complains of severe epigastric pain. On examination there is abdominal guarding and rigidity.

1) a.
Invagination of loose scrotal skin allows palpation of the inguinal canal through the external ring. A lump above and medial to the pubic tubercle is an inguinal hernia. To differentiate between an indirect and a direct inguinal hernia place your finger on the internal ring (located 1 cm above the femoral pulse at the midinguinal point) and ask the patient to cough. A lump below and lateral to the pubic tubercle is a femoral hernia.

2) c.
This occurs when a dilatation of the long saphenous vein occurs at its junction with the femoral vein in the groin.

3) c.
This patient has cauda equina syndrome. The most common cause of this condition is a prolapsed intervertebral disc. Other causes include tumour, trauma and infections.

4) e.
The patient would be fed via nasogastric tube or percutaneous endoscopic gastrostomy (PEG).

5) a.
Diabetes is a complication of chronic pancreatitis.

6) d.
Major operations, in particular orthopaedic surgery, are a risk factor for developing DVT and PE.

7) b.
This is prophylactic treatment against pulmonary embolism.

8) c.
This is a rare autosomal dominant condition causing development of benign polyps within the GI system.

9) a.
Then notify the surgical registrar of your findings.

10) d.
Calot's triangle consists of the lower edge of the liver superiorly, the common hepatic duct medially and the cystic duct inferiorly. It contains the cystic artery and Calot's lymph node. During laparoscopic cholecystectomy, it is important to dissect out Calot's triangle so as to visualize the structures and avoid biliary damage.

11) b.

12) e.
A large-bore needle is preferable (14G) and should be inserted in the second intercostal space just above the third rib to avoid nerves and blood vessels that run just beneath the ribs.

13) c.
Once haemodynamically stable, the patient will require an urgent endoscopy.

14) e.

15) b.
The oral contraceptive pill can cause mastalgia itself.

16) a.
Composition of the lump can be determined as well as analysis of any fluid aspirated.

17) b.
Steroids are a risk factor for peptic ulcer formation.

18) a.
This will show free air under the diaphragm. Free air under the diaphragm is almost always due to a perforated hollow viscus.

19) c.
Small areas of calcium deposits in the breast are known as breast calcifications and are divided into macrocalcifications and microcalcifications. Macrocalcifications are usually harmless. Microcalcifications are seen in areas of the breast with a high cell turnover. A cluster of microcalcifications can be a sign of breast cancer.

20) a.
This can be due to a number of reasons: a low cardiac output, underlying atherosclerotic disease or use of vasopressors during surgery.

21) c.
This is the gold standard tool and can be used for both diagnosis and treatment of the condition.

22) c.

23) a.
The axillary nerve supplies the deltoid muscle, which abducts the shoulder. Injury to the axillary nerve also causes a loss of sensation in the upper lateral arm – the regimental badge area.

24) d.
Primary chemotherapy is used to shrink inoperable breast tumours to make them amenable to surgery.

25) b.
Follicular thyroid carcinoma implies capsular invasion, which cannot be diagnosed on FNAC. Frozen section is required at hemithyroidectomy.

26) b.
Adrenal atrophy is a complication of steroid therapy.

27) c.
Ultrasonography is used to determine the diameter of the aortic aneurysm. If the diameter is >5.5 cm, there is increased risk of rupture and AAA repair is advocated.

28) b.
Seminomas are radiosensitive.

29) a.
Facial nerve palsy with a parotid mass on the same side is pathognomonic of parotid malignancy.

30) e.

31) c.
A sigmoidoscopy allows visualization of the last 60 cm of the colon whereas a colonoscopy visualizes the entire colon (up to 152 cm), allowing any possible neoplasm to be detected.

32) b.
This shows loss of abductor pollicis brevis function.

33) e.
Indicating acute cholangitis.

34) b

35) c.
Ultrasonography has a 95% sensitivity for gallstones that are >2 mm. Ultrasonography is unreliable in picking up stones in the common biliary duct or cystic duct. A HIDA scan is used if gallstone disease is suspected but not demonstrated on an ultrasound scan.

36) d.
Thiazide diuretics are associated with hypercalcaemia. Loop diuretics are associated with increased calcium excretion.

37) e.

38) d.
This is the gold standard because it directly visualizes the thrombus and is useful if non-invasive tests, such as ultrasonography, have failed to discover a strongly suspected DVT.

39) e.
Other causes of postoperative renal failure include nephrotoxic medications, underlying medical disorders and the nature of the surgery itself.

40) e.
The common causes of postoperative fever can be summarized in the following mnemonic: wind (atelectasis, pneumonia), wound, water (UTI), walking (DVT/PE) and wonder drugs. Atelectasis is a common cause of pyrexia in the early post-surgery period.

41) a.
This patient has a bowel ileus and has aspirated into the right lower lobe of the lung.

42) b.
Mesenteric ischaemia is a well-known complication of AAA repair. The diagnosis should be considered if the patient presents with diarrhoea and abdominal pain in the postoperative period.

43) a.
An ABG (arterial blood gas) will quickly assess the level of oxygenation to the tissues.

44) b.
Another, although less common, condition is the fat embolism syndrome where trauma or surgery to large long bones or the pelvis can cause numerous fat droplets to enter the circulation with widespread systemic effects.

45) c.
Whipple's operation is offered to patients with masses in the head of the pancreas. The head of the pancreas, a portion of the bile duct, the gallbladder and the duodenum are removed. Part of the stomach may also be removed.

46) c.
FNA is less invasive than a Tru-Cut biopsy so it can be carried out while the patient is in outpatients. FNA can also be used to distinguish between a cystic and a solid lump.

47) d.

48) a.

49) a.

50) c.
This is a complication of ulcerative colitis and is life threatening. The colon needs to be decompressed (nil by mouth and nasogastric tube) to prevent perforation and aggressive fluid resuscitation is crucial. If there is no improvement a colectomy should be considered.

51) e.
Loperamide may precipitate a paralytic ileus and megacolon.

52) b.
A cut over a knuckle is presumed to be a human bite until proven otherwise. Human bite wounds should be left open to heal. Antibiotics are indicated to cover for anaerobic streptococci.

53) c.

54) e.

55) c.

56) c.
Chemotherapy is effective on cancer cells that divide rapidly such as breast and colorectal carcinomas. Prostatic carcinomas grow slowly and divide at the same rate as healthy cells, hence chemotherapy is not usually successful.

57) e.
Increased levels of glucose are the usual finding in burn victims. This is due to high levels of circulating glucocorticoids and increased insulin resistance.

58) e.
Loss of haustral markings in the colon on the radiograph is seen in ulcerative colitis.

59) a.
This patient has compartment syndrome.

60) c.
There is no benefit in having the procedure.

61) e.
Poorer prognosis is associated with BANS (back, back of arms, neck and scalp), trunk and ulcerated malignant melanomas.

62) b.
The urine in sterile pyuria contains a very large number of WBC ($>10/mm^3$) and appears sterile using standard culture techniques. TB should be considered and three early morning urine samples should be sent to the laboratory for culture.

63) e.
This patient has a pelvic fracture with a urethral injury.

64) b.

65) e.
Liver failure results in depleted glycogen stores and consequently causes hypoglycaemia.

66) a.
This patient has a pharyngeal pouch. The signs and symptoms are classic and the pouch may be palpable on the left side of the neck.

67) c.

68) d.
Although gas may be seen in the soft tissues of the neck and around the mediastinum on plain films, a water-based contrast swallow will also localize the perforation. The patient may also have subcutaneous emphysema.

69) c.

70) c.
This sign can be seen in acute appendicitis.

71) e.

72) d.
The neck of a femoral hernia is narrow and more likely to incarcerate.

73) b.

74) c.
A stone may have inadvertently moved in to the CBD intraoperatively. Typical features of cholangitis would be fever, abdominal pain and jaundice.

75) a.

76) b.
The risk of recurrence after curative surgery for colonic cancer is significantly raised if a preoperative blood transfusion is administered. This is thought to be due to the immunosuppressive blood components that promote tumour growth.

77) e.

78) c.
TURP syndrome may occur if the operation is prolonged, i.e. > 1 h, and if excessive fluid irrigation is used.

79) e.

80) c.

81) e.
PET is not readily available in all hospitals.

82) d.
Most cases of adhesions are due to previous abdominal surgery.

83) b.
Pethidine injections provide fast and effective analgesia in severe pain. Diclofenac is used in mild-to-moderate cases of pain.

84) a.
Percutaneous nephrostomy is used to relieve renal obstruction.

85) b.
Cefuroxime is the antibiotic of choice for orthopaedic surgery with prosthetic material.

86) c.
Metronidazole as required is advised 4 hours preoperatively in an appendectomy.

87) d.

88) d.
Vancomycin is indicated to cover *Staphylococcus aureus* and coagulase-negative staphylococci.

89) e.

90) a.
The Balthazar score (also known as the CT severity index) assesses the severity of inflammation and necrosis in pancreatitis.

91) c.
D-dimers are a product of fibrinolysis and occur as part of the breakdown products of a blood clot.

92) d.
Antimuscarinic agents are used in the treatment of urinary frequency.

93) c.
Avascular necrosis is a common complication as the blood supply is easily interrupted by the fracture.

94) b.

95) e.

96) d.
A thromboembolus in the carotid arteries accounts for over 80% of transient ischaemic attacks (TIAs).

97) b.
Erosion of the anterior wall and into the innominate artery can result in catastrophic bleeding and death.

98) d.
Hyperkalaemia is a complication of massive blood transfusions.

99) a.

100) e.

101) b.
Intrinsic factor is found in the stomach and is important in vitamin B_{12} absorption. Gastrectomy patients require supplementation to prevent pernicious anaemia.

102) e.
The patient should be treated for hypercalcaemia secondary to malignancy.

103) d.
Signs of venous hypertension should be checked, not arterial insufficiency.

104) d.

105) a.
Perianal abscesses arise from an infection of the anal glands, and people with diabetes and Crohn's disease are more susceptible. Incision and drainage lead to immediate symptomatic relief.

106) b.
Gas gangrene is one of the indications for a below-knee amputation. Other indications include trauma, malignancy and gangrene as a result of peripheral vascular disease.

107) c.

108) a.
Tumours that commonly metastasize to bone are thyroid, breast, bronchus, prostrate and kidney tumours. Prophylactic fixation of impending fractures is also beneficial and should be considered in patients who present with pain at a known site of metastasis.

109) c.

110) e.
Carotid body tumours are located in the anterior triangle of the neck and present as a painless slow-growing lump in the neck. They are rare and usually benign lesions found at the bifurcation of the carotid artery. Surgical removal is advocated to prevent compression of neurovascular structures.

111) b.
The middle meningeal artery is at risk from trauma to the temporal bone of the skull.

112) d.

113) c.
This patient has sustained a urethral injury. Insertion of a Foley catheter is contraindicated due to the possibility of converting a partial tear of the urethra into a complete tear.

114) b.

115) e.
The patient is shocked and not stable enough for a CT scan. Take the patient directly to theatre.

116) e.

117) e.
Vocal fold palsy causes airway obstruction because the folds fix in a closed position at the entrance to the trachea.

118) e.
Laparoscopic surgery supersedes open cholecystectomy as the first choice of treatment for gallstone disease. The bowel is not manipulated as much during keyhole surgery as during open surgery so postoperative ileus is rare.

119) d.
Other initial investigations for jaundice include clotting screen, FBC, inflammatory markers and U&Es. Ultrasound scanning and MRCP (magnetic resonance cholangiopancreatography) should be considered before ERCP, which is an invasive procedure.

120) a.
In this procedure the endoscope is passed via the mouth into the duodenum. The muscular valve at the ampulla of Vater is dissected (papillotomy) to allow the extraction of bile duct stones from the lower end of the duct via a balloon catheter.

121) b.

122) c.
In this patient, obstruction of the superior vena cava (SVC) is most likely due to an apical lung cancer.

123) b.
This operation involves incising the thickened pylorus muscle to form a larger gastric outlet and therefore relieve the obstruction.

124) c.
This condition – testicular torsion – is often misdiagnosed as epididymo-orchitis, so beware!

125) d.

126) b.
This man has angiodysplasia. As the colonic mucosa is not distorted, a barium enema is not useful; it also causes visual difficulties for other diagnostic modalities.

127) d.
Angiodysplasias are dilatations of blood vessels in the GI mucosa, which bleed easily due to their fragility. On colonoscopy the lesions are seen as small, flat, 'cherry-red' areas.

128) c.
This woman has acute diverticulitis with peritoneal signs and requires urgent laparotomy.

129) a.
Dukes' stage A is associated with a 90% 5-year survival rate, Dukes' stage B 60–70% and Dukes' stage C 30–60% at 5 years.

130) d.
Dupuytren's contracture is associated with liver disease.

131) e.
Cholangiocarcinomas are adenocarcinomas of the biliary tree. They are rare and occur more commonly in Asia due to parasitic infestations. Less than 15% of tumours are resectable and palliative measures, such as insertion of percutaneous stents, are the mainstay of treatment.

132) a.
This man has stigmata of alcohol liver disease and portal hypertension.

133) e.

134) a.

135) b.
Sclerosing cholangitis is a condition in which there is inflammation and fibrosis of the intra- and extrahepatic bile ducts, which can lead to cirrhosis.

136) c.

137) c.
'Pus somewhere, pus nowhere, pus under the diaphragm.' Be alert when confronted with a patient with a persistent swinging pyrexia of unknown origin, occurring several days postoperatively. There is usually a hidden abscess or, in this case, a subphrenic abscess.

138) a.

This man most likely requires blood replacement because a lengthy operation is often associated with greater blood loss.

139) c.

Blood group A and not O is associated with stomach cancer. Sister Mary Joseph's sign is the association of a hard umbilical nodule with poorer prognosis for intra-abdominal malignancy (i.e. sign of gastric carcinoma metastasis). She was Dr William Mayo's surgical assistant.

140) b.

Causes of carpal tunnel syndrome include hypothyroidism, pregnancy, obesity, rheumatoid arthritis and acromegaly.

141) e.

142) e.

CEA is elevated in patients with colorectal cancer. This tumour marker can be used to check disease activity and the effect of treatment.

143) c.

Fracture of the scaphoid bone causes pain and tenderness in the anatomical snuffbox — the hollow between the base of the thumb and wrist. Scaphoid views should be taken on radiograph if such a fracture is suspected.

144) e.

Blood group A is associated with stomach cancer and not oesophageal cancer.

145) e.

In a tension pneumothorax, the trachea is shifted to the contralateral side, causing obstruction to the venous return to the heart and consequently cardiorespiratory arrest.

146) d.

The first two ribs are the hardest to break.

147) d.

A widened mediastinum is defined as mediastinal widening of >8 cm on a supine chest radiograph. Causes include aortic dissection, retrosternal thyroid and tumours.

148) b.
This patient needs urgent referral to a specialist hospital centre because cardiopulmonary bypass is required for thoracic aortic arch repair. Leave the specialist centre to organize the CT scan. If it is normal, the centre can always send the patient back to you. You will not have lost any time.

149) a.

150) b.

151) e.
Before 1950, the most common site was the antrum, but, with the rise in cancer of the lower oesophagus and gastric cardia, 40% of adenocarcinomas are found in the fundus and cardia. Radical gastrectomy is offered for stages I–III.

152) b.
This patient should receive palliative care due to the terminal nature of his condition.

153) b.
Acute respiratory distress syndrome occurs either due to direct lung injury or due to severe underlying illness. Indications for ventilation include PaO_2 <8.3 kPa despite 60% O_2 and $PaCO_2$ >6 kPa.

154) c.
Intravenous opiates should be administered for analgesia.

155) c.
Endoscopy allows both diagnosis and treatment of an upper GI bleed. Angiography should be considered in patients in whom endoscopy has failed and in those in whom surgery is considered high risk.

156) e.
Endoscopic intubation is a procedure used to introduce an endotracheal tube under direct visual control via an endoscope.

157) d.
The bacterium spreads haematogenously from a distant focus of infection to infect the metaphysis of long bones. *Staphylococcus aureus* causes osteomyelitis in over 90% of cases.

158) e.

159) a.

The BNF guidelines state that 7 days of triple therapy is adequate to eradicate 90% of cases of *Helicobacter pylori*. Any longer and patient compliance is poor due to the side effects of the medications. Heliclear comes prepackaged, containing these drugs. Helimet is an alternative that includes lansoprazole (proton pump inhibitor), clarithromycin and metronidazole.

160) e.

161) e.

Prostaglandins are produced within cells by the enzyme cyclo-oxygenase (COX-1 and COX-2). Both these enzymes produce prostaglandins, which cause inflammation, pain and fever. COX-1 also produces prostaglandins that support platelets and protect the stomach. NSAIDs block both these COX enzymes and reduce prostaglandins throughout the body so that inflammation, pain and fever are reduced. As the prostaglandins that protect the stomach and blood clotting are also reduced, NSAIDs can cause ulcers in the stomach and promote bleeding.

162) c.

The abscess can be drained percutaneously during ultrasonography or CT.

163) e.

164) c.

165) c.

Further investigations are focused on locating metastases.

166) d.

Studies involving the ingestion of caustic substances indicate that there is no benefit in the use of steroids to prevent stricture formation.

167) a.

168) e.

169) a.

This patient has a positive Pemberton's sign. Raising her arms above her head decreases the size of the thoracic inlet and worsens symptoms.

170) a.

Pemberton's sign is indicative of an obstruction to the SVC due to a retrosternal goitre, lung cancer (especially apical), lymphomas or other mediastinal masses.

171) b.

172) d.

173) a.

The patient presents with an acute thrombus at the site of the femoral artery.

174) a.

175) e.

Colonoscopy allows full visualization of the colon up to the terminal ileum, which is affected in a large proportion of patients with Crohn's disease.

176) e.

Hypoparathyroidism due to inadvertent removal or injury to the parathyroid glands during thyroidectomy can lead to low serum calcium. Other complications of this operation include recurrent laryngeal nerve palsy, hypothyroidism and tracheal obstruction from haematoma formation.

177) a.

The single-celled protozoan causes gastrointestinal symptoms, in particular watery diarrhoea, flatulence, abdominal cramps and nausea. Giardiasis is spread via the faecal–oral route and most people become infected by drinking contaminated water.

178) d.

Metronidazole is the treatment of choice in giardiasis. It inhibits certain liver enzymes which break down the by-product of ethanol, acetaldehyde. A build-up of acetaldehyde causes flushing, tachycardia, headache and nausea.

179) d.

A mallet finger occurs when there is injury to the extensor tendon of the distal phalanx. The patient cannot actively straighten the joint but can do so passively.

180) c.
Malignant hyperthermia is reported to occur in 1 in 50 000 anaesthetics. The condition is inherited in an autosomal dominant manner. Symptoms include muscle rigidity, fever, tachycardia, renal failure and cardiac arrhythmias.

181) d.

182) a.
Exposure to the anaesthetic agent causes an abnormal rise in intracellular calcium. The subsequent sustained muscle contraction leads to an increase in ATP and oxygen consumption and heat production. Cell damage occurs and leakage of potassium and myoglobin causes the clinical picture.

183) d.
The biceps nearly always ruptures at the long head and occurs after a long period of tendonitis. On examination the muscle bunches up in the upper arm, resulting in the 'Popeye' biceps appearance.

184) b.

185) b.
Anticoagulation with warfarin requires several days to achieve a therapeutic effect, so heparin is used immediately and simultaneously to prevent clot enlargement.

186) c.

187) a.
Poor wound healing from uraemia is due to a general reduction in cell proliferation, particularly of collagen and granulation tissue. Patients also tend to suffer from anaemia, which also contributes to poor healing.

188) b.
Approximately 75% of pancreatic cancers occur in the head and neck of the pancreas. Peak age of incidence is 60–80 years and only 20% are amenable to surgery at the time of diagnosis.

189) d.
Oesophageal perforation due to excessive vomiting is known as Boerhaave's syndrome and is classically seen in those with a recent intake of large amounts of alcohol or food. Oesophageal rupture from

any cause (iatrogenic, trauma, foreign body inhalation, repeated episodes of emesis) is a surgical emergency. Management is with immediate surgical repair, intravenous antibiotics and fluids.

190) c.
This is a genetic disorder in which abnormally high levels of iron are absorbed through the intestine and are deposited in various organs around the body.

191) b.

192) b.
Froment's sign is used to test the competence of the ulnar nerve. A piece of paper is placed between the thumb and upturned palm. The patient is asked to hold on to the paper while it is being pulled away. Flexion at the distal interphalangeal joint of the thumb occurs as a compensatory action because the adductor pollicus, supplied by the ulnar nerve, is paralysed.

193) c.

194) c.
Undisplaced and stable fractures can be strapped to the adjacent finger to minimize misalignment.

195) e.
This patient has a hip fracture of which intertrochanteric fractures are the most common, especially in elderly patients.

1) A.
Classic presentation for acute appendicitis.

2) G.
Gallstones and alcohol are the main predisposing factors for acute pancreatitis.

3) H.
Chronic active hepatitis is associated with methyldopa and also isoniazid.

4) L.
A large proportion of diverticula occurs in the sigmoid colon. They are associated with poor dietary intake.

5) J.
This is an uncommon complication of total hip replacement and usually occurs in elderly patients. Co-morbidities, poor mobility and high analgesia requirements also contribute to the condition.

6) F.
Axillary lymphadenopathy is indicative of malignancy.

7) B.

8) E.
The most important diagnosis to exclude here is breast cancer, which can be done only on biopsy.

9) J.
Paget's disease or intraductal carcinoma is associated with eczema of the nipple, especially in the presence of a firm nodule suggestive of more than simple eczema.

10) H.
Risk factors for a breast abscess include diabetes, immunosuppression, smoking and mastitis.

11) I

12) D.
A thyroglossal cyst moves on swallowing or protrusion of the tongue.
The fact that the swelling transilluminates excludes a thyroid swelling.

13) F.
The swelling would present in the lateral side of the neck and can result
from tooth infections and middle-ear infections.

14) A.
By the end of the fourth week of gestation, five branchial (pharyngeal)
arches have developed, which form different structures of the head,
neck and thorax. A branchial cyst arises from remnants of the branchial
arch, which has not completely obliterated.

15) B.
Ludwig's angina, a submandibular abscess, usually arises from an
abscess of the lower premolars or the first and second molars.

16) D.

17) I.
Diamorphine is three times more powerful than morphine and is
administered in a syringe driver so as to provide continuous pain relief.

18) G.

19) H.
NSAID use may precipitate an asthma attack.

20) C.

21) B.
Chvostek's sign is demonstrated here and is associated with
hypocalcaemia.

22) A.
An upright chest radiograph would show free air under the diaphragm
due to a perforated peptic ulcer secondary to anti-anginal medication.

23) J.
Blood loss from a hip fracture often warrants blood replacement.

24) H.
Pulmonary embolism is suggested here.

25) I.
Epidural anaesthesia may be associated with urinary retention.

26) H.
The presentation is suggestive of ureteric colic.

27) I.
The presentation is suggestive of an ovarian cyst.

28) C.
The presentation is suggestive of peptic ulcer disease.

29) A.
The presentation is suggestive of abdominal aortic aneurysm. The size should be evaluated by ultrasonography and surgical repair is advisable if the aneurysm is >5.5 cm in diameter.

30) K.
Steroid usage for rheumatoid arthritis puts this woman at risk of a perforated peptic ulcer.

31) A.
Presbyacusis is confirmed by a pure-tone audiogram, which would demonstrate symmetrical high-frequency sensorineural hearing loss.

32) D.
Syringing, cotton bud usage and swimming are recognized risk factors for otitis externa.

33) I.
A conductive hearing loss with a normal tympanic membrane is suggestive of otosclerosis.

34) E.
Chronic secretory otitis media or glue ear is treated with watchful waiting for 3 months. If spontaneous resolution has not occurred, referral to an ENT specialist may be necessary.

35) H.
This patient has a false-negative Rinne test, suggestive of a dead ear.

36) H.
This is infection of the nailfold.

37) K.

38) C.
Opinion is divided as to whether acromegaly causes carpal tunnel syndrome by compression of the median nerve by bony enlargement and soft-tissue swelling or due to swelling of the nerve itself.

39) A.
This is a well-known and dreaded complication of supracondylar fractures. It results from injury or compression to the brachial artery; if the blood supply is not restored within a 6- to 8-hour period then function is lost.

40) E.
Smoking, caffeine ingestion and stress can aggravate symptoms in Raynaud's phenomenon.

41) D.
These tears usually occur at the gastro-oesophageal junction and occur after forceful, prolonged vomiting.

42) K.

43) C.
This patient has developed portal hypertension secondary to cirrhosis.

44) E.

45) F.
Virchow's node is associated with stomach cancer and on examination may be the only sign of an intra-abdominal malignancy.

46) I.
Courvoisier's law states that, 'if, in a case of painless jaundice, the gallbladder is palpable, the cause will not be gallstones'.

47) K.
This is a rare benign tumour that can occur anywhere along the GI mesentery.

48) A.
Acute appendicitis is less likely without nausea and Crohn's ileitis is less likely without diarrhoea.

49) G.
Carcinoma of the caecum is associated with bleeding.

50) E.

The most common presentation of carcinoma of the sigmoid is changes in bowel habit rather than pain.

51) C.

Beck's triad consists of muffled heart sounds, hypotension and Kussmaul's sign, and is pathognomonic for cardiac tamponade.

52) G.

53) M.

Absence of the psoas shadow is due to retroperitoneal fluid.

54) I.

55) K.

Addisonian crisis is precipitated here by omission of doses of a long-term steroid regimen.

56) B.

In a fit man aged under 60, AO cannulated screws are preferable to an Austin Moore hemiarthroplasty. In elderly people a hemiarthroplasty is favoured because they can mobilize while healing is under way.

57) F.

Anterior cruciate ligament injury should be repaired surgically, especially in a young athlete.

58) I.

Dynamic hip screw is the standard treatment for intertrochanteric fractures.

59) D.

Scapholunate disassociation is repaired by open reduction of the subluxation and a K wire to hold the reduction. The wrist is then splinted.

60) K.

Anterior shoulder fracture–dislocation requires open reduction and fixation.

61) I.

Dysphagia, stridor, dysphonia and an expanding neck haematoma are all indications to explore a penetrating neck wound.

62) H.

63) C.
Prompt insertion of a needle or chest tube into the left pleural space is indicated to relieve the pneumothorax.

64) I.
Immediate surgical exploration is warranted. An on-table angiogram can be obtained simultaneously.

65) I.
Traumatic diaphragmatic rupture is associated with deceleration injuries and requires prompt surgical exploration.

66) J.
Pseudocysts usually arise as a complication of pancreatitis.

67) K.
Divarication of the rectus abdominis muscles is associated with multiple pregnancies and chronic abdominal distension. The gap is palpable on examination.

68) I.
Spontaneous splenic rupture after minor blunt trauma is associated with infectious mononucleosis.

69) B.
Bleeding oesophageal varices are often the cause of massive haematemesis in children.

70) B.
This patient has underlying liver disease causing portal hypertension and oesophageal varices.

71) A.
Malignant hyperthermia may be precipitated by halothane or suxamethonium.

72) B.
Chvostek's sign is a sign of hypocalcaemia, which may occur after thyroidectomy and injury to the parathyroid glands.

73) E.
Aspiration pneumonia may occur in a patient with postoperative ileus, drowsiness or altered swallowing.

74) I.
This patient is in urinary retention.

75) K.
This patient may need blood replacement.

76) H.
Diaphragmatic rupture can be diagnosed on chest radiograph by the presence of bowel or the nasogastric tube being seen in the chest.

77) G.
This usually arises from chest injury sustained by hitting the steering wheel with great force.

78) C.

79) I.
Open pneumothorax is treated by covering the wound with a piece of gauze that is taped down along three sides to act as a flutter valve.

80) D.
Kussmaul's sign is a classic sign for cardiac tamponade, as is Beck's triad. However, not all patients present with the classic signs!

81) K.
A Glasgow Coma Scale (GCS) score of 3 is the lowest score possible.

82) J.
A GCS of 8 or less and absence of a gag reflex are both indications for intubation.

83) F.
No mention of airway management has been made and therefore should be included in the initial assessment of this patient.

84) F.
Penetrating objects should be left *in situ* until surgery. Again airway assessment is always the first priority in management of head injuries.

85) G.
Hypotension should not be assumed to be caused by brain injury.

86) C.
Acute back strain is treated conservatively.

87) F.
Night pain and pathological fractures should make one suspicious for underlying pathology.

88) G.
Acute cauda equina syndrome requires urgent decompression.

89) D.
Mechanical back pain is treated conservatively.

90) H.
Intervertebral disc prolapse is the most common cause of root pain.

91) A.
Battle's sign (bruising over the mastoid process), raccoon eyes (periorbital bruising), haemotympanum and CSF leak in the ears or nose are all signs associated with basal skull fracture.

92) F.

93) E.
Concussion is the transient loss of consciousness without accompanying neurological signs.

94) H.

95) C.
If the dura was breached, the diagnosis is one of open skull fracture.

96) A.

97) C.
Surgical repair is undertaken in athletes or for associated rotator cuff tears.

98) D.
Painful arc syndrome is treated with injections of local anaesthetic and steroids. The syndrome is due to degenerative changes of the supraspinatus tendon.

99) A.
Acromioclavicular joint subluxation or dislocation is treated conservatively with a broad arm sling followed by mobilization.

100) G.
The Hippocratic technique is a one-man technique as opposed to Kocher's manoeuvre which requires an assistant for counter-traction. Pain may be a limiting factor to successful reduction.

101) F.
The plantar fascia runs from the calcaneum to the heads of the metatarsals. It acts as a shock absorber and reinforces the arch of the foot. Injuries to the fascia from excessive activities can cause inflammation and therefore pain articularly near the calcaneum.

102) G.
Avascular necrosis of the head of the second metatarsal is thought to be the cause of Freiberg's disease. Avascular necrosis occurs from microstress fractures at the junction of the metaphysis and growth plate, leading to a reduced blood supply at the epiphysis.

103) A.
Longstanding irritation of the interdigital nerves, which run between the metatarsals, can cause thickening of part of the nerve. It commonly affects the nerve between the third and fourth metatarsals.

104) B.
A bone scan may be necessary to confirm a stress fracture.

105) D.

106) A.
Hypertension will contribute to ongoing epistaxis. Nifedipine is advisable to lower the patient's BP. She will then need to see her GP for regular antihypertensive therapy.

107) K.
Any patient on warfarin who presents with epistaxis should have the clotting screen checked. Treatment with vitamin K may be required. However, the haematologist should be consulted for advice if this is the case.

108) F.
A food bolus containing bone is at high risk for perforating the oesophagus and needs prompt attention.

109) G.
This patient can be managed conservatively at first with Buscopan, a muscle antispasmodic. She will need an outpatient barium swallow on discharge.

110) **D.**
This patient will need a sialogram if the parotid swelling reoccurs.

111) **A.**
A chest radiograph may show air in the soft tissues but a Gastrografin swallow is conclusive in the diagnosis of oesophageal perforation.

112) **E.**

113) **G.**
A technetium scan should be arranged to investigate for Meckel's diverticulum.

114) **F.**

115) **H.**

116) **F.**
Medical therapy should be initiated. Mesalazine is a newer aminosalicylate that avoids the side effects of sulfasalazine.

117) **E.**
The liver and spleen are at high risk of injury from blunt trauma to the abdomen.

118) **C.**
Acute cholecystitis is managed conservatively until an urgent ultrasound scan can be arranged.

119) **A.**

120) **D.**
This patient has toxic megacolon and is at high risk of perforation when the transverse diameter of the colon exceeds 6 cm.

121) **D.**
Proctalgia fugax results from spasm of the anal sphincter and often occurs at night with episodes lasting a few minutes.

122) **F.**

123) A.

A tear of the anal canal causes intense pain especially on defecation. A fissure *in ano* should be suspected if pain is out of proportion on per rectum exam.

124) E.

Constipation, pregnancy, heavy lifting and long periods of sitting down are all predisposing factors.

125) G.

126) G.

Pleural effusions due to malignancy are most commonly caused by carcinomas of the breast, ovary, lung, gastrointestinal tract or by lymphomas. In this patient an ascetic tap will yield fluid that should be sent to the laboratory for investigations to include cytology analysis.

127) D.

IV fluids (for hydration and renal calcium clearance), loop diuretics (increases calcium excretion and prevents fluid overload) and bisphosphonates (reduces osteoclastic activity) are used in the treatment of hypercalcaemia.

128) F.

This is an emergency and surgical decompression is required to prevent irreversible paralysis.

129) A.

Approximately 20% of breast cancer patients will develop brain metastases.

130) B.

This patient has bony metastatic disease which has caused weak bone structure.

131) H.

The spleen is the most commonly injured organ in blunt trauma. The capsule surrounding this organ allows slow bleeding with subsequent shock when the capsule ruptures.

132) E.

Other radiological findings for aortic rupture include widened mediastinum, a pleural apical cap, tracheal displacement to the right, multiple rib fractures and depression of the left main stem bronchus.

133) I.

Other radiological findings include bowel loops in the chest and curling of the nasogastric tube in the chest.

134) B.

Surgery is indicated if extravasation of dye is observed on CT as this indicates pelvic avulsion.

135) J.

3. PSYCHIATRY

3. Psychiatry: SBA/BOF Questions

In these questions candidates must select one answer only.

1) A 70-year-old woman requests to be started on an antidepressant for a 1-year history of depression. She also has a history of poorly controlled epilepsy. The most suitable medication to start with is:

   a. Donepezil
   b. Dothiepin
   c. An MAOI (monoamine oxidase inhibitor)
   d. Sertraline (an SSRI – selective serotonin reuptake inhibitor)
   e. Venlafaxine

2) A 40-year-old man is diagnosed with schizophrenia. The most appropriate first-line outpatient medication to initiate is:

   a. Citalopram
   b. Haloperidol
   c. Chlorpromazine
   d. Olanzapine
   e. Piportil Depot

3) You suspect that one of your patients, a 16-year-old girl, is suffering from an eating disorder. The physical finding that best supports your suspicion is:

   a. Nystagmus
   b. Weight loss
   c. Anaemia
   d. Froment's sign
   e. Erosion of tooth enamel and abrasions on dorsal aspects of fingers

4) The following drugs are a recognized treatment for bipolar disorder EXCEPT:

   a. Sodium valproate
   b. Lithium
   c. Carbamazepine
   d. SSRIs
   e. Phenytoin

5) A 55-year-old homeless man is brought to A&E. The police are concerned for his welfare. On examination, he is unkempt with dirty fingernails and talks very quietly. He hesitates briefly before he responds appropriately to your questions. His face does not change expression. The most likely diagnosis is:

a. Depression
b. Schizophrenia
c. Parkinson's disease
d. Hypothyroidism
e. Temporal lobe epilepsy

6) Appropriate initial investigations for this man include all of the following EXCEPT:

a. FBC
b. TFTs
c. Urine toxicology
d. Calcium and glucose
e. EEG

7) Immediate side effects of antipsychotic drugs include all of the following EXCEPT:

a. Tardive dyskinesia
b. Dystonias
c. Oculogyric crisis
d. Neuroleptic malignant syndrome
e. Akathisia

8) Which of the following evidence-based questionnaires is used for postnatal depression?

a. Hamilton
b. Beck
c. Edinburgh
d. MAST
e. CAGE

9) A 40-year-old inpatient being treated for paranoid schizophrenia threatens to leave the hospital. Under which Section of the Mental Health Act 1983 can he be detained by you as a junior doctor?

a. 2
b. 3
c. 4
d. 5
e. 7

10) A 30-year-old woman is brought to A&E by the police under Section 136 of the Mental Health Act 1983 for self-neglect. Under which Section can she then be admitted and detained for 72 hours?

a. 2
b. 3
c. 4
d. 5
e. 12

11) A 40-year-old woman has been grieving for 18 months for her deceased child. She is both depressed and anxious all the time. Appropriate management includes all of the following EXCEPT:

a. SSRIs
b. Benzodiazepines
c. Cognitive–behavioural therapy
d. Buspirone
e. EMDR (eye movement desensitization and reprocessing)

12) A 20-year-old woman complains of recurrent episodes of chest tightness, paraesthesiae and difficulty breathing. The episodes peak in severity within 10 min. After exclusion of any physical aetiology, appropriate management includes all of the following EXCEPT:

a. Breathing into a paper bag
b. Tricyclic antidepressant
c. Cognitive–behavioural therapy
d. An SSRI
e. An MAOI

13) A 20-year-old woman presents with chest pain. She is wearing baggy trousers and an oversized jumper. You suspect anorexia nervosa. Her height is 1.5 m and her weight is 36 kg. Her body mass index (BMI) is:

a. 15
b. 16
c. 17
d. 20
e. 24

14) A 55-year-old woman complains of depression for 6 months. She has lost interest in sex and food, and has insomnia. Appropriate investigations include all of the following EXCEPT:

a. Prolactin
b. FBC
c. Glucose
d. TFTs
e. LFTs

15) A 35-year-old man has complained of auditory hallucinations and his family report that he has become more socially withdrawn. The following statement is true regarding schizophrenia:

   a. The risk of suicide is approximately the same as that for the general population
   b. There is no benefit to social rehabilitation therapies
   c. Early use of antipsychotics alters the course of the illness
   d. There is no genetic predisposition
   e. Cannabis use has not been implicated

16) A 55-year-old man who suffers from alcoholism is hospitalized for acute alcoholic hepatitis. The liver unit would like you to start alcohol detoxification. The most appropriate drug to use is:

   a. Heminevrin (chlormethiazole)
   b. Diazepam
   c. Acamprosate
   d. Disulfiram
   e. Lofexidine

17) A 20-year-old man who is an intravenous drug abuser requests drug therapy. He injects 1.5 g heroin daily and uses two rocks a week. The first step in management is to:

   a. Take urine for toxicology to confirm presence of opiates
   b. Take blood for FBC and LFTs
   c. Take blood for hepatitis B and C and HIV test
   d. Commence methadone at 20 mL daily on a daily pick-up basis
   e. Commence buprenorphine therapy at an initial dose of 4 mg

18) A 25-year-old man is brought to A&E obtunded. He has no physical signs of head trauma. He has needle marks on his neck and groin. His pupils are pinpoint. His respiratory rate is 6/min. He is receiving 100% oxygen by facemask and an anaesthetist is present. The next most immediate management would be:

   a. Urine for toxicology
   b. Naloxone injection
   c. Endotracheal intubation
   d. Flumazenil antidote
   e. Arterial blood gas

19) A 55-year old man admitted for alcohol detoxification suddenly starts fitting in front of you on the ward. The initial treatment for status epilepticus is:

   a. Rectal diazepam
   b. Intramuscular diazepam
   c. Intravenous diazepam
   d. Intravenous phenytoin sodium
   e. Rectal paraldehyde

20) A 40-year-old man who was a passenger in a serious RTA complains of flashbacks, hypervigilance, insomnia and poor concentration. Recognized treatment includes all of the following EXCEPT:

a. EMDR
b. Antidepressants
c. β Blockers
d. Relaxation therapies
e. CBT

21) High-risk indicators for suicide include all of the following EXCEPT:

a. Being male
b. Family history of suicide
c. Drug abuse
d. Depression
e. Age <40 years

22) Schneider's symptoms of the first rank suggestive of the diagnosis of schizophrenia include all of the following EXCEPT:

a. Delusional perception
b. Somatic passivity
c. Flat affect
d. Thought block
e. Third-person auditory hallucinations

23) A 23-year-old woman presents with a history of catastrophic mood swings, and intense and multiple relationships; she describes her life as emotional chaos. She has cut herself in the past to relieve emotional pain. She drinks alcohol and indulges in cannabis. Her family states that she has always been like this and likens her to a 2 year old having a tantrum. The most likely diagnosis is:

a. Bipolar disorder
b. Borderline personality disorder
c. Schizotypal disorder
d. Antisocial personality disorder
e. Histrionic personality disorder

24) A 40-year-old patient has been on fluoxetine for 3 months and asks when he should discontinue the medication, as he is feeling much better now. You advise him to continue for:

a. 1 month
b. 6 weeks
c. 3 months
d. 6 months
e. 1 year

25) Side effects of tricyclic antidepressants include all of the following EXCEPT:

a. Postural hypotension
b. Drowsiness
c. Agranulocytosis
d. Convulsions
e. Cardiotoxicity

26) A 70-year-old woman on dothiepin, a tricyclic antidepressant, presents with convulsions. The most useful blood test is:

a. FBC
b. INR
c. LFTs
d. Sodium
e. Potassium

27) A 40-year-old woman complains that she has had no response to fluoxetine 20 mg once daily for her depression after 8 weeks. She also complains of chronic anxiety and insomnia. The next line of drug for depression would be:

a. Venlafaxine
b. An MAOI
c. Benzodiazepine
d. A tricyclic antidepressant
e. Moclobemide

28) Appropriate measures in dealing with aggressive patients include all of the following EXCEPT:

a. Lower the pitch of your voice
b. Keep your hands in full view of the patient
c. Be punctual
d. Sit facing the patient
e. Position yourself closer to the door

29) Physical disorders that may mimic anxiety include all of the following EXCEPT:

a. Carcinoid syndrome
b. Alcohol intoxication
c. Excessive caffeine
d. Thyrotoxicosis
e. Hypoglycaemia

30) A 40-year-old woman complains of several months of anxiety, insomnia, irritability and depression following an acrimonious divorce. She requests medication to help her sleep. Appropriate treatment may include all of the following EXCEPT:

   a. Short-term benzodiazepine
   b. Referral for counselling
   c. Buspirone
   d. SSRI
   e. A β blocker

31) A 50-year-old man reports consuming the equivalent of 36 units of alcohol a week. The most appropriate screening test for problem drinking is:

   a. CAGE
   b. γ-Glutamyltransferase
   c. Mean corpuscular volume
   d. The presence of spider naevi
   e. The presence of a tender liver edge

32) A 45-year-old man reports feeling increasingly low and finds it difficult to find pleasure in anything. Which of the following symptoms most increases his risk for suicide:

   a. Tearfulness
   b. Sleep disturbance
   c. Anorexia
   d. Lethargy
   e. Feelings of hopelessness

33) Alcohol consumption is associated with all of the following EXCEPT:

   a. 80% of suicides
   b. Half of all hospital admissions
   c. 40% of RTAs
   d. 80% of deaths from fire
   e. One in three cases of child abuse

34) A 40-year-old man with longstanding schizophrenia now presents with fever and impaired consciousness. On examination there is muscle rigidity, a labile blood pressure and tachycardia. Serum creatine kinase is raised. The most likely diagnosis is:

   a. Septicaemia
   b. Tardive dyskinesia
   c. Neuroleptic malignant syndrome
   d. Acute myocardial infarction
   e. Meningitis

35) A 55-year-old man is taking lithium for bipolar disorder. In addition to checking the blood levels of lithium, the following tests should be arranged every 3 months EXCEPT for:

a. LFTs
b. TFTs
c. FBC
d. ECG
e. U&Es

36) A 20-year-old woman states that she is usually up all night doing one thing or another. She describes herself as a very busy woman with lots of new and exciting projects. She gets annoyed with her family for being obstructive to some of her plans. She admits to shopping excessively. Her family reports that she has always been a busy bee. What is the most likely diagnosis?

a. Borderline personality disorder (emotionally unstable)
b. Anankastic (obsessional) personality
c. Bipolar disorder
d. Obsessive–compulsive disorder
e. Drug or alcohol addiction

37) A 45-year-old woman describes a fear of being contaminated with industrial chemicals. She reports that she is showering longer and longer every evening in an attempt to remove these chemicals. She knows that this is an irrational fear. The following neurotransmitter is implicated in this condition.

a. Acetylcholine
b. Serotonin
c. Dopamine
d. Noradrenaline
e. Glutamate

38) Features of heroin withdrawal syndrome include all of the following EXCEPT:

a. Insomnia
b. Muscle cramps
c. Diarrhoea
d. Yawning
e. Pinpoint pupils

39) Complications produced by intravenous drug abuse include all of the following EXCEPT:

a. Hepatitis C
b. Deep vein thrombosis
c. Hepatitis A
d. Thrombophlebitis
e. Cellulitis

40) Features of benzodiazepine withdrawal syndrome include all of the following EXCEPT:

   a. Anxiety
   b. Hallucinations
   c. Tinnitus
   d. Heightened sensitivity to light
   e. Pinpoint pupils

41) Drug treatments for Alzheimer's disease include all of the following EXCEPT:

   a. Donepezil
   b. Lovasatatin
   c. Galantamine
   d. Rivastigmine
   e. Selegiline

42) Characteristic features of dementia include all of the following EXCEPT:

   a. Abrupt onset
   b. Aggressive outbursts
   c. Decrement in memory and judgement
   d. Poor social and personal relationships
   e. Clear consciousness

43) Reversible causes of dementia include all of the following EXCEPT:

   a. Hypothyroidism
   b. Hypoparathyroidism
   c. Communicating hydrocephalus
   d. Vitamin B$_{12}$ deficiency
   e. Renal failure

44) Negative symptoms of schizophrenia include all of the following EXCEPT:

   a. Poverty of thought
   b. Blunted affect
   c. Auditory hallucinations
   d. Social withdrawal
   e. Poverty of speech

45) Potential side effects of atypical antipsychotics include all of the following EXCEPT:

   a. Weight loss
   b. Agranulocytosis
   c. Hepatitis
   d. Extrapyramidal symptoms
   e. Postural hypotension

46) Features of schizophrenia include all of the following EXCEPT:

a. Ambivalence
b. Loosening of associations
c. Paranoia
d. Loss of affect
e. Excessive anxiety

47) You are called to the ward to see a 45-year-old, acutely disturbed patient. He cannot be calmed. You decide that he requires rapid tranquillization. He has no history of heart disease. The nurses restrain the patient while you inject which medication?

a. Droperidol 10 mg i.m. + lorazepam 2 mg i.m.
b. Depot antipsychotic (Piportil Depot) i.m.
c. Zuclopenthixol acetate 100–150 mg i.m.
d. Chlorpromazine 25 mg i.m.
e. Morphine 10 mg i.v.

48) Components of the Mini-Mental State Examination (MMSE) include all of the following EXCEPT:

a. Speech
b. Appearance
c. Diagnosis
d. Perception
e. Intellect

49) Side effects of tricyclic antidepressants include all of the following EXCEPT:

a. Bradycardia
b. Weight gain
c. Dry mouth
d. Disturbance of eye accommodation
e. Increased intraocular pressure

50) A 60-year-old man with schizophrenia requires compulsory admission to hospital for treatment of his disorder. Under which Section of the Mental Health Act 1983 should he be admitted for treatment?

a. 2
b. 3
c. 4
d. 5
e. 7

51) Features of childhood autism include all of the following EXCEPT:

   a. Abnormal response to pain
   b. Imitation
   c. Echolalia
   d. Avoidance of mutual gaze
   e. Impaired imagination

52) Features of delirium include all of the following EXCEPT:

   a. Clouding of consciousness
   b. Gradual, stepwise onset
   c. Perseveration
   d. Delusions
   e. Labile mood

53) Strategies in long-term psychotherapy include all of the following EXCEPT:

   a. Reflecting
   b. Linking
   c. Free association
   d. Confrontation
   e. Paternalism

54) Indications for electroconvulsive therapy may include all of the following EXCEPT:

   a. High suicide risk
   b. Psychotic depression
   c. Depression unresponsive to antidepressants
   d. Post-traumatic stress disorder
   e. Depression with marked psychomotor retardation

55) Medical presentations of alcoholism include all of the following EXCEPT:

   a. Memory loss
   b. Gastritis
   c. Pancreatitis
   d. Hypertension
   e. Carcinoma of the prostate

56) Complications of delirium tremens include all of the following EXCEPT:

   a. Hypothermia
   b. Dehydration
   c. Convulsions
   d. Chest infection
   e. Electrolyte imbalance

57) Organic causes of mania include all of the following EXCEPT:

a. HIV infection
b. Malaria
c. Hypothyroidism
d. Cerebral tumour
e. SLE

58) Medium duration (weeks) side effects of antipsychotic drugs include all of the following EXCEPT:

a. Amenorrhoea
b. Impotence
c. Prolonged Q–Tc interval
d. Weight gain
e. Tardive dyskinesias

59) Features of mania may include all of the following EXCEPT:

a. Flight of ideas
b. Pressure of speech
c. Irritability
d. Evident in early life
e. Grandiose beliefs

60) A 65-year-old woman develops mild confusion, disorientation and anxiety postoperatively after the administration of high doses of analgesia. The best course of management would be:

a. Soft restraints to the bed
b. Adequate doses of a benzodiazepine for sedation
c. A darkened room with decreased sensory stimulation
d. A well-lit room with frequent interaction
e. Administration of haloperidol

61) A 20-year-old, slightly withdrawn man states that he experiences auditory hallucinations. He is noted to have poverty of speech and a flat affect. The most likely diagnosis would be:

a. Schizophrenia
b. Bipolar disorder
c. Delirium
d. Dementia
e. Opioid abuse

62) Diagnostic features of post-traumatic stress disorder include all of the following EXCEPT:

a. Autonomic arousal
b. Recurrent, obtrusive thoughts
c. Symptoms of anxiety
d. Memory impairment
e. Loss of orientation

63) Diagnostic features of panic disorder include all of the following EXCEPT:

a. Dizziness
b. Feelings of unreality
c. Fear of insanity
d. Fear of leaving home
e. Choking sensations

64) Diagnostic features of mania include all of the following EXCEPT:

a. Labile mood
b. Rapid speech
c. Loss of inhibitions
d. Overeating
e. Grandiosity

65) The following are symptoms of schizophrenia EXCEPT:

a. Obsessional intrusive thoughts
b. Thought insertion
c. Poverty of speech
d. Suspiciousness
e. Primary delusion

66) The following conditions can mimic panic disorder EXCEPT:

a. Phaeochromocytoma
b. Hyperthyroidism
c. Hypoglycaemia
d. Caffeine withdrawal
e. Barbiturate withdrawal

67) A 20-year-old man presents for psychotherapy. He is manipulative and lacks empathy. He has a grandiose sense of self-importance and entitlement. The most likely personality disorder would be described as:

a. Antisocial
b. Borderline
c. Histrionic
d. Schizotypal
e. Narcissistic

68) The average age of onset of schizophrenia is:

a. 15–25
b. 25–35
c. 35–45
d. 45–55
e. >60

69) The following are first-rank symptoms of schizophrenia EXCEPT:

a. Anhedonia
b. Bodily sensations being imposed by an outside agency
c. Delusional perceptions
d. Third-person auditory hallucinations
e. Alien thoughts

70) Risk screen for danger to others includes the presence of the following EXCEPT:

a. Morbid jealousy
b. Hallucinations giving instructions
c. Thought disorder
d. Lack of remorse about past history of violence
e. Violent fantasies

71) Treatment of longstanding anxiety include the following, EXCEPT:

a. Venlafaxine
b. Fluoxetine
c. Sertraline
d. Diazepam
e. Citalopram

72) The following statements regarding obsessive–compulsive disorder are correct, EXCEPT:

a. Females and males are equally affected
b. Depression is unusual
c. Obsessional thoughts are recognized by patients as being their own
d. Obsessional thoughts are usually pleasant in nature
e. Over 60% of cases have improved at the end of 1 year

73) An 8-year-old boy has nocturnal enuresis. Investigations reveal no underlying conditions. The most appropriate treatment is:

a. Analytical psychotherapy
b. Behavioural therapy
c. Counselling
d. Crisis therapy
e. Problem-solving

74) St John's wort can be used in the treatment of:
   a. Schizophrenia
   b. Obsessive–compulsive disorder
   c. Anxiety
   d. Depression
   e. Bipolar disorder

75) The number of units in a bottle of vodka is:
   a. 1
   b. 10
   c. 20
   d. 25
   e. 32

3. Psychiatry: EMQ Questions

Theme: treatment of psychiatric conditions

Options

A. Buprenorphine (Subutex)
B. Mirtazapine
C. Amitriptyline
D. Chlordiazepoxide
E. Carbamazepine
F. Olanzapine
G. An SSRI
H. Lofexidine
I. Heminevrin (chlormethiazole)
J. Electroconvulsive therapy
K. Haloperidol
L. Sodium valproate
M. Lithium
N. Venlafaxine
O. Acamprosate

For each patient below, choose the SINGLE most likely treatment from the list of options. Each option may be used once, more than once or not at all.

1) A 30-year-old man who is an intravenous drug abuser asks for heroin detoxification therapy. He has tried a methadone regimen of 30 mL once daily without success and would like to try something new. His urine screen confirms the presence of heroin, methadone and cocaine.

2) A 50-year-old man with alcohol problems requests alcohol detoxification therapy. You refer him to a local community inpatient detox centre. Which drug will he be given?

3) A 20-year-old woman complains of depression lasting for 1 year. You evaluate her depression as moderate. Which drug would you start her on?

4) A 30-year-old man presents with obtrusive auditory hallucinations that tell him to kill himself. He informs you that he will not harm himself. Which medication would you consider commencing?

5) A 55-year-old man requests medication to help him resist alcohol. He has completed an alcohol detox programme. Which drug would you start him on?

Theme: diagnosis of psychiatric disorders

Options

A. Suicidal risk
B. Alcohol abuse
C. Generalized anxiety
D. Dementia
E. Panic attacks
F. Bipolar disorder
G. Drug abuse
H. Depression
I. Delirium
J. Grief reaction
K. Schizophrenia
L. Borderline personality disorder

For each patient below, choose the SINGLE most likely diagnosis from the list of options. Each option may be used once, more than once or not at all.

6) A 70-year-old retired engineer experiences changes in personality and impaired social skills. This is corroborated by his family, who describe him as forgetful and not as sharp as he used to be.

7) A 20-year-old man is noted to be withdrawn, isolated and 'peculiar'. He experiences persecutory delusions and auditory hallucinations. His urine toxicology screen is clear.

8) A 60-year-old widow is noted by her family to be restless, disorganized and crying, and frequently expresses her wish to join her deceased partner.

9) A 40-year-old Irishman complains of frequent episodes of chest pains, sweating, palpitations, a sense of impending doom and paraesthesiae that last for minutes at a time.

10) A 25-year-old man presents with miosis, slurred speech, disorientation and respiratory depression.

Theme: treatment of psychiatric disorders

Options

A. Long-term psychotherapy
B. Lithium
C. Donepezil
D. Levodopa
E. Diazepam
F. Risperidone
G. Tetrabenazine
H. Propranolol
I. Disulfiram
J. Methadone
K. Fluoxetine

For each case below, choose the SINGLE most appropriate treatment from the list of options. Each option may be used once, more than once or not at all.

11) A 70-year-old man presents with progressive forgetfulness and mood changes. He has a shuffling gait. A CT scan of the head shows cortical atrophy and enlarged ventricles.

12) A 60-year-old man presents with a disturbance of voluntary motor function. His face is expressionless. On examination cogwheel rigidity and bradykinesia are present.

13) A 10-year-old boy presents with brief, repetitive motor tics and is brought in by his parents for shouting obscenities at school.

14) A 40-year-old man presents with ataxia. His wife states that it runs in her husband's family. He is difficult to live with, very irritable and clumsy, and has jerky movements of the legs.

15) A 20-year-old man presents with sweating, muscle twitching and abdominal cramps. On examination his pupils are dilated.

Theme: diagnosis of organic mental disorders

Options

A. Parkinson's disease
B. Huntington's disease
C. Alzheimer's disease
D. Multi-infarct dementia
E. Creutzfeldt–Jakob disease
F. Korsakoff's psychosis
G. Temporal lobe seizures
H. Wernicke's encephalopathy
I. Chronic subdural haematoma
J. Subarachnoid haemorrhage
K. Acute intermittent porphyria

For each patient below, choose the SINGLE most likely diagnosis from the list of options. Each option may be used once, more than once or not at all.

16) A 70-year-old man presents with gradual deterioration of memory and intellect. His family has noticed a change in personality and behaviour.

17) A 35-year-old man presents with dementia and choreiform movements.

18) A 60-year-old man with alcohol dependence presents with deterioration of both retrograde and anterograde memory. He invents stories.

19) A 60-year-old man with alcohol dependence presents with persistent headache. His family notes that he is inattentive and becoming more confused.

20) A 65-year-old man presents with an abrupt onset of confusion and ataxia. On examination, nystagmus is present. He is a known drinker.

Theme: diagnosis of psychiatric disorders

Options

A. Schizophrenia
B. Brief reactive psychosis
C. Bipolar disorder
D. Major depression
E. Body dysmorphic disorder
F. Panic disorder
G. Post-traumatic stress disorder
H. Schizoaffective disorder
I. Delusional disorder
J. Paranoid schizophrenia
K. Postpartum depression
L. Dysthymia

For each patient below, choose the SINGLE most likely diagnosis from the list of options. Each option may be used once, more than once or not at all.

21) A 40-year-old man insists that his wife is unfaithful and sleeping with the entire neighbourhood. He is hypersensitive, argumentative and litigious. His wife has left him due to his behaviour. He functions well at work.

22) A 25-year-old woman presents with personality changes. She is noted by friends initially to be anxious and irritable, and an insomniac; weeks later she becomes profoundly depressed with low self-esteem and contemplates suicide. In consultation she has pressured speech with boundless energy.

23) A 20-year-old woman has a 'mental breakdown'. She has recently broken up with her boyfriend. She has dramatic mood swings, memory loss and incoherent speech. This lasts for a month.

24) A 20-year-old woman presents to her GP complaining of feeling depressed ever since she can remember. Her parents died in a car crash 10 years ago. She sees herself as a failure, but functions well at work. She has trouble falling asleep.

25) A 50-year-old woman complains of sudden episodes of impending doom. During these episodes she feels like she is choking and sweats profusely.

Theme: diagnosis of psychiatric conditions

Options

A. Pica
B. Formication
C. Alcohol withdrawal
D. Alcohol intoxication
E. Schizophrenia
F. Xenophobia
G. Agoraphobia
H. Algophobia
I. Delirium
J. Fugue
K. Cocaine intoxication
L. Opioid withdrawal
M. Drug toxicity

For each patient below, choose the SINGLE most likely diagnosis from the list of options. Each option may be used once, more than once or not at all.

26) A 3-year-old boy presents with anaemia and abdominal pain. His mother states that she has seen him peeling paint chips off the wall and wonders if he has been eating these.

27) A 23-year-old woman becomes afraid to leave her home. She functions normally except that she will not step outside her house.

28) An 18-year-old man presents with nausea, vomiting and diaphoresis. He has dilated pupils. Blood pressure is elevated. He has a history of drug addiction.

29) A 30-year-old woman is found in an amnestic state. Her husband reports that she had been missing for a few days after she had been served with divorce papers.

30) A 30-year-old man takes lithium for longstanding bipolar disorder. He was recently started on thiazide diuretics for mild hypertension and is now confused with ataxia, blurred vision and a coarse tremor.

Theme: diagnosis of psychiatric disorders

Options

A. Munchausen's syndrome
B. Alcohol withdrawal delirium
C. Extrapyramidal side effects
D. Hypothyroidism
E. Hysterical neurosis
F. Acromegaly
G. Dissociative disorder
H. Malingering disorder
I. Parkinson's disease
J. Cushing's syndrome
K. Autonomic side effects of drug
L. Anticholinergic side effects of drug

For each patient below, choose the SINGLE most likely diagnosis from the list of options. Each option may be used once, more than once or not at all.

31) A 28-year-old woman presents with lower abdominal pain. On examination there are multiple surgical scars over her abdomen. Abdominal and pelvic examinations are normal. She insists that she needs a laparoscopy.

32) A 50-year-old man with schizophrenia is started on haloperidol. A month later he is noted to be drooling saliva and walking with a shuffling gait. He also suffers from involuntary chewing movements.

33) A 40-year-old woman complains of dry mouth, blurry vision and constipation. On examination she has dilated pupils. She was started on amitriptyline for major depression.

34) A 45-year-old man complains of headaches, excessive thirst and frequent urination. On examination he is noted to have bad acne, coarse skin and a goitre. He has moved his wedding band to the fifth finger.

35) A 30-year-old man presents to A&E with a dislocated shoulder. On examination the shoulder is found not to be dislocated. The patient insists that it is dislocated, and he needs morphine for the pain.

Theme: management of psychiatric disorders

Options

A. Benzodiazepine medication
B. Cognitive–behavioural therapy
C. Depot antipsychotic
D. Electroconvulsive therapy
E. Antidepressant medication
F. Psychotherapy
G. Referral to occupational therapist

For each of the presentations below, choose the SINGLE most appropriate management from the list of options. Each option may be used once, more than once or not at all.

36) A 30-year-old woman is moderately depressed with no suicidal ideation. She does not want to start antidepressant medication at the moment.

37) A 28-year-old man has frequent hallucinations, delusions and arguments with his neighbours. He has been unresponsive to olanzapine and does not pick up his prescription on a regular basis.

38) A 21-year-old man has become progressively withdrawn over the last few weeks. He has told his girlfriend that he has bought six packets of paracetamol and wants to end his life. He is absolutely adamant about his statement.

39) A 35-year-old man is admitted to hospital with acute schizophrenia. He is experiencing frightening persecutory delusions. Two days later he becomes very agitated and begins to threaten staff and patients.

40) A 55-year-old man with chronic schizophrenia is to be discharged from hospital; the hostel is concerned about the risks of his being left alone while preparing food.

Theme: diagnosis of psychiatric disorders

Options

A. Acute confusional state
B. Post-traumatic stress disorder
C. Personality disorder
D. Obsessive–compulsive disorder
E. Generalized anxiety disorder
F. Psychosis
G. Borderline personality disorder
H. Mania
I. Depressive episode

For each of the presentations below, choose the SINGLE most appropriate diagnosis from the list of options. Each option may be used once, more than once or not at all.

41) A 40-year-old man undergoes surgery for a fractured humerus. Three days after the operation, he becomes agitated and confused, and has tremors. He says that he can see pink elephants.

42) A 30-year-old Afghani refugee has been complaining of nightmares since he came to the UK 18 months ago. He becomes highly startled at the slightest of noises.

43) A 45-year-old woman comes into the surgery. You note her restlessness and how she talks about one topic and jumps shortly to another.

44) A 45-year-old woman complains of poor concentration and memory over the last few months. She says that she is bound to lose her job and will become destitute. She is adamant that a serious physical disease is causing her problems.

45) A 34-year-old man comes in to the surgery concerned that a stranger whom he had seen in the street the day before has forcibly entered his flat during the night. He called the police in a very agitated state but they found no sign of entry. His brother with whom he lives says that he is behaving very strangely and seems rather paranoid.

1) d.
Donepezil is a reversible acetylcholinesterase inhibitor that acts on the CNS. Its main use is in Alzheimer's disease. Dothiepin (also known as dosulepin) is a TCA; this class of antidepressant has the highest risk of seizures. SSRIs (first-line treatment for depression) and venlafaxine (second-line treatment) are the agents of choice in epilepsy. MAOIs, although safe, are limited by their side-effect profile.

2) d.
Newer atypical antipsychotics are now a recognized first-line therapy for schizophrenia preferred to typical antipsychotic agents such as haloperidol and chlorpromazine.

3) e.
Self-induced vomiting can cause erosion of tooth enamel by exposure to gastric acid. Finger abrasions develop from repeated insertion of fingers into the throat, which scratch against the teeth.

4) e.

5) b.
This patient is displaying negative symptoms of schizophrenia.

6) e.
Initial investigations are directed towards eliminating other possible causes for this patient's symptoms such as infection, drug abuse and biochemical abnormalities. EEG is recommended for patients in whom various treatment measures have failed; it is particularly effective if catatonia is also present.

7) a.
Tardive (delayed/late-appearing) dyskinesia (movement difficulties) occurs after long-term use of antipsychotic drugs.

8) c.
Scores >13 indicate depression.

9) d.
The Mental Heath Act was introduced in 1983 and allows detainment (also known as sectioning) of patients with possible mental illness

who may harm themselves or others. Section 2 admits the patient for assessment for up to 28 days. Section 3 admits the patient for treatment for up to 6 months. Section 4 allows emergency admission for up to 72 hours. Voluntary patients on the wards can be detained by a doctor under Section 5(2) or by a nurse under Section 5(4).

10) c.
Section 136 allows the police to remove someone from a public place who appears to have a mental disorder, and take them to a 'place of safety' for assessment and/or treatment. A place of safety is usually a hospital, police station or specialist residential home for patients with psychiatric disorders.

11) e.
EMDR is a recognized treatment for post-traumatic stress disorder and helps resolve traumatic memories.

12) e.

13) b.
Body mass index $=$ weight (kg)/height (metres)^2.

14) a.

15) c.
Research shows that a better outcome is seen in patients with early use of antipsychotics and the maintenance of social skills. Rates of suicide are almost nine times more than among the general population. Cannabis has been implicated in the onset of schizophrenia. There is a definite genetic predisposition for the condition, shown by adoptive studies.

16) b.
Heminevrin is no longer recommended as attenuation therapy for alcohol dependence because there is a high risk of mortality if consumed with alcohol.

17) a.
Urinalysis is the most common method of drug analysis. Other methods include the testing of hair, blood, saliva and sweat.

18) b.
Naloxone is a competitive antagonist for centrally located opioid receptors.

19) c.
Intravenous diazepam should be administered ideally in a setting with access to resuscitation equipment.

20) c.
This patient is suffering from PTSD.

21) e.
Age >40 years is a risk factor for suicide.

22) c.

23) b.

24) d.
Antidepressants should be continued for 6−9 months after the patient's mood improves.

25) c.
Agranulocytosis is a side effect of antipsychotic medication.

26) d.
Hyponatraemia is associated with tricyclic antidepressants, especially in the elderly population.

27) a.
Venlafaxine is a drug that treats both anxiety and depression, and so would be useful in this patient's case.

28) d.
Sitting sideways to the patient is less confrontational.

29) b.
Symptoms of alcohol intoxication include slurred speech, incoordination, ataxia, nystagmus and respiratory depression.

30) e.

31) a.
Men should limit their alcohol intake to 3−4 units/day and women to 2−3 units/day. In the UK, the driving limit is 80 mg alcohol per 100 mL blood, which is approximately 2 pints of regular lager.

32) e.

33) b.
Of all hospital admissions 10–30% are associated with alcohol.

34) c.
This life-threatening condition arises from a reaction to antipsychotic medication. It is due to the blockade of dopamine receptors within the corpus striatum causing muscle rigidity, fever and altered consciousness.

35) a.
Side effects of lithium include hypothyroidism, hypokalaemia, raised ADH, ECG changes and renal changes.

36) c.

37) b.
This patient has OCD. Serotonin is thought to be implicated in OCD because SSRIs are a highly effective class of medication.

38) e.
Dilated pupils are associated with opiate withdrawal.

39) c.
Hepatitis A is transmitted by the faecal–oral route.

40) e.

41) e.
Selegiline is used in the treatment of Parkinson's disease

42) a.

43) b.
Hyperparathyroidism and not hypoparathyroidism is a reversible cause of dementia.

44) c.
Third-person auditory hallucination is a positive symptom of schizophrenia.

45) a.
Weight gain is a recognized side effect of antipsychotics and can increase the risk of non-compliance, diabetes and heart disease.

46) e.

47) a.

48) c.

49) a.
Tachycardia is a side effect of TCAs.

50) b.
Section 3 allows the patient to be detained in hospital for treatment. It typically follows a Section 2, which allows the patient to be detained in hospital for assessment.

51) b.
In autism, imitation is impaired.

52) b.
Delirium is an acute confusional state.

53) e.

54) d.
Patients with a high suicide risk may require ECT as antidepressants take 2 weeks to produce an effect.

55) e.

56) a.
Hyperthermia and not hypothermia is associated with delirium tremens

57) e.

58) e.
Long-term use of antipsychotic medication, as well as high dosages, can cause movement disorders.

59) d.
Personality disorders are evident in early life.

60) d.
This is a case of delirium caused by analgesics. This reaction is common in hospitalized older patients. As well as treating the underlying cause, she should receive supportive measures such as frequent interaction and help with orientation. Darkness and restraint further agitate delirious patients.

61) a.

62) e.

63) c.

64) d.

65) a.
These are a feature of obsessive–compulsive disorder.

66) d.
Caffeine intoxication and not withdrawal may mimic panic disorder.

67) e.

68) a.

69) a.
Anhedonia is the inability to gain pleasure from normally pleasurable activities. It is seen in depression, schizophrenia and other mental illnesses. but is not classed as a first rank symptom of schizophrenia.

70) e.

71) d.
Diazepam should not be given for more than 2–4 weeks as addiction to and dependence on the drug can develop within this time frame.

72) d.
Obsessional thoughts are unpleasant; some common thoughts include the fear of contamination, fear of leaving doors unlocked and fear of harming someone.

73) b.
This is the single most effective treatment for this condition. It involves the use of a bedwetting alarm that is triggered when moisture is detected. The child then wakes and should empty the bladder in the toilet.

74) d.
This is a herbal antidepressant.

75) e.

3. Psychiatry: EMQ Answers

1) A.
Subutex is a long-acting opioid that binds to opiate receptors in the brain; its pleasurable effects are much less pronounced than those of other opiates such as heroin, so it is used to prevent withdrawal symptoms in a patient who is detoxing.

2) D.
This is a long-acting benzodiazepine that is used in alcohol detox on a dose-reducing regimen.

3) G.
An SSRI such as fluoxetine or paroxetine could be prescribed.

4) F.
An atypical antipsychotic would be the first choice.

5) O.
Research shows that this drug is effective if support groups are attended at the same time.

6) D.

7) K.

8) A.
Patients who have lost a partner are not routinely prescribed antidepressants but encouraged to experience a grief reaction. However, this woman does not have a typical grief reaction, as she has expressed a wish to join her partner. She should be assessed for risk of suicide and asked if she has made plans.

9) E.

10) G.

11) C.
This is a reversible inhibitor of acetylcholinesterase, used in the treatment of Alzheimer's disease.

12) D.
Levodopa is used in combination with a dopa-decarboxylase inhibitor. This inhibitor prevents the metabolism of levodopa to dopamine within the periphery and therefore allows more dopamine to penetrate the blood–brain barrier to act on the corpus striatum.

13) F.
Risperidone is used to reduce the vocal and motor tics associated with Gilles de la Tourette's syndrome.

14) G.
Tetrabenazine is used in the treatment of chorea in Huntington's disease.

15) J.
Methadone is used in heroin detoxification; it prevents the unpleasant symptoms experienced in drug withdrawals.

16) C.
One of the earliest signs of Alzheimer's disease is memory loss.

17) B.

18) F.
This results from thiamine deficiency and arises if Wernicke's encephalopathy is left untreated.

19) I.

20) H.
Wernicke's encephalopathy describes a syndrome of mental confusion, ataxia and ophthalmoplegia.

21) I.

22) C.

23) B.

24) L.

25) F.

26) A.
Pica is the ingestion of non-food substances such as clay and dirt.

27) G.

28) K.

29) J.
Fugue states are usually triggered by stressful events and are defined as a temporary episode of action followed by complete amnesia for the time of the activity. The activity usually involves the patient travelling unexpectedly away and becoming confused about his or her identity. These episodes of fugue can last hours, months or even years.

30) M.
Thiazide diuretics increase the secretion of sodium ions. As a result co-administration with lithium can cause higher concentrations of lithium because fewer sodium ions are available for lithium clearance by the renal system.

31) A.

32) C.
Extrapyramidal side effects are caused by antidopaminergic agents, particularly haloperidol. Management is to switch to an atypical antipsychotic (clozapine, risperidone) or to reduce the current dose.

33) L.
TCAs have antimuscarinic, anticholinergic side effects; they have largely been replaced by SSRIs as first-line therapy for depression.

34) F.
In most cases the excessive production of growth hormone is the result of a pituitary adenoma.

35) H.

36) B.
Research shows that CBT is highly effective in treating depression and anxiety disorders. Higher rates of response are seen with a combination of CBT and antidepressant medication than by either therapy alone.

37) C.
Depot antipsychotics are administered intramuscularly so that the drug is released over several weeks. Depots can be used to promote treatment compliance and adherence.

38) D.
Antidepressants take at least 2 weeks to produce a clinical result. This patient has severe major depression and ECT produces far more rapid results than antidepressants.

39) A.
Benzodiazepines are a useful adjunct in the acute phase of schizophrenia to control agitation.

40) G.

41) A.
This patient is suffering from alcohol withdrawal.

42) B.

43) H.

44) I.

45) F.

4. OBSTETRICS AND GYNAECOLOGY

4. Obstetrics and Gynaecology: SBA/BOF Questions

In these questions candidates must select one answer only.

1) In which circumstance is rhesus immunization NOT required in a rhesus-negative mother?

   a. Following amniocentesis
   b. After delivery of a rhesus-negative baby
   c. After a threatened miscarriage at 10 weeks' gestation
   d. After termination of pregnancy at 8 weeks' gestation
   e. After a spontaneous miscarriage at 12 weeks' gestation

2) Endometrial cancer is associated with all of the following EXCEPT:

   a. Combined oral contraceptive pills
   b. Premarin (HRT) use in postmenopausal women with a uterus
   c. Early menopause
   d. Hypothyroidism
   e. Multiple pregnancy

3) Routine blood tests offered at a booking antenatal clinic include all of the following EXCEPT:

   a. HIV antibody test
   b. Serology for hepatitis B
   c. Haemoglobin electrophoresis in a pregnant woman from India
   d. FBC
   e. Clotting studies

4) Increased serum human chorionic gonadotrophin (hCG) is associated with each of the following EXCEPT:

   a. Choriocarcinoma
   b. Hyperemesis gravidarum
   c. Pregnancy
   d. Ovarian carcinoma
   e. Hydatidiform mole

5) Cervical smear may suggest the diagnosis of all of the following EXCEPT:

   a. Adenomyosis
   b. Bacterial vaginosis
   c. *Trichomonas vaginalis*
   d. CIN
   e. Invasive carcinoma of the cervix

6) The following statements regarding the Mirena coil are correct EXCEPT:

   a. It contains levonorgestrel
   b. It controls menorrhagia
   c. It needs to be changed every 5 years
   d. It is not advisable in women with a past history of PID
   e. It increases the absolute risk of ectopic pregnancy

7) Postcoital bleeding can occur with each of the following EXCEPT:

   a. Cervical polyp
   b. CIN
   c. *Trichomonas vaginalis* infection
   d. Cervical ectropion
   e. Endometrial carcinoma

8) Deep dyspareunia can occur with each of the following EXCEPT:

   a. Pelvic inflammatory disease
   b. Ovarian neoplasm
   c. Ectopic pregnancy
   d. Bartholin's abscess
   e. Endometriosis

9) Intermenstrual bleeding may be associated with each of the following EXCEPT:

   a. Subserous fibroids
   b. Polycystic ovarian syndrome
   c. Carcinoma of the cervix
   d. Combined oral contraceptives
   e. Intrauterine contraceptive device

10) Appropriate investigations for a 32-year-old woman 5 days after an emergency caesarean section who now presents with per vagina bleeding and passage of blood clots include all of the following EXCEPT:

   a. Transvaginal ultrasound scan
   b. FBC
   c. Vaginal swab for microscopy and culture
   d. LFTs
   e. Clotting studies

11) Causes of preterm labour include all of the following EXCEPT:

   a. Chorioamnionitis
   b. Polyhydramnios
   c. Cervical incompetence
   d. Human papillomavirus
   e. Pyelonephritis

12) Complications of pre-eclampsia include all of the following EXCEPT:

   a. IUGR
   b. Renal failure
   c. Thrombocytopenia
   d. Cerebrovascular accident
   e. Hypoglycaemia

13) A 20-year-old woman is diagnosed with polycystic ovarian syndrome. She does not plan to conceive in the near future. Which treatment would you offer this patient?

   a. Cyproterone acetate (Dianette)
   b. Clomiphene citrate
   c. Wedge resection of the ovaries
   d. Microgynon (combined oral contraceptive pill)
   e. Zoladex

14) Causes of dysmenorrhoea include all of the following EXCEPT:

   a. Endometriosis
   b. IUCD (intrauterine contraceptive device)
   c. Pelvic inflammatory disease
   d. Subserosal fibroids
   e. Polycystic ovarian disease

15) The following statements regarding ectopic pregnancy are correct EXCEPT:

   a. Risk factor includes the IUCD
   b. It occurs in 1 in 200 pregnancies
   c. It may present with shoulder-tip pain
   d. It never presents with bilateral lower abdominal pain
   e. It may be treated with injection of methotrexate into the unruptured ectopic

16) Appropriate forms of contraception after delivery for a mother who plans to breastfeed include all of the following EXCEPT:

   a. Implanon
   b. Progestogen-only pill
   c. Depo-Provera
   d. IUCD
   e. Combined oral contraceptive pill

17) The differential diagnosis for postmenopausal bleeding includes all of the following EXCEPT:

   a. Carcinoma of the cervix
   b. Adenomyosis
   c. Endometrial polyp
   d. Atrophic vaginitis
   e. Endometrial carcinoma

18) A 14-year-old girl complains of dysmenorrhoea. She states that she is not sexually active. The most appropriate medication would be:

a. Tranexamic acid
b. Mefenamic acid
c. Paracetamol
d. Microgynon
e. Fluoxetine

19) Management of menorrhagia may include all of the following EXCEPT:

a. Norethisterone tablets 5 mg three times daily for 10 days
b. Tranexamic acid 1 g three times daily for 3 days
c. Placement on the combined oral contraceptive pill
d. Insertion of the Mirena intrauterine system
e. Zoladex

20) A 20-year-old woman requests emergency contraception. She had unprotected sexual intercourse 48 hours ago and has not been using any form of contraception. She has never been pregnant. Her LMP was 16 days ago. What would you offer her?

a. Combined oral contraceptive pill
b. Levonelle
c. Mirena coil
d. Depo-Provera
e. Implanon

21) You are summoned by the midwife to see Mrs Elliot who has just had a spontaneous vaginal delivery. She is lying in a pool of blood. The following steps in management are correct EXCEPT:

a. Insert two large-bore Venflons and take blood for FBC, clotting, and type and cross-match (T+C) 2 units
b. Alert the obstetric registrar, senior midwife and anaesthetist
c. Rub the uterus and check the placenta for tears
d. Commence Syntocinon infusion
e. Consent the patient for examination under anaesthesia

22) A 50-year-old woman presents with worsening urinary incontinence over the past 2 years. She has had three spontaneous vaginal deliveries (SVDs) and is now menopausal. She is not taking any medication. She states that the symptoms are worse when she coughs or sneezes. No prolapse is noted on pelvic examination. The following investigations are appropriate EXCEPT:

a. Urine dipstick for glucose and MSU for microscopy and culture
b. FBC and U&Es
c. Pelvic ultrasonography
d. Uroflowmetry
e. Cystometry

23) A 28-year-old obese woman presents with difficulty in conceiving. She also complains of deep pelvic pain, dysmenorrhoea and deep dyspareunia. Her cycles come every 21 days and last for 10 days. The most likely diagnosis is:

a. Polycystic ovarian disease
b. Endometriosis
c. Ovarian remnant syndrome
d. Chronic PID
e. Fibroid uterus

24) A 27-year-old woman complains of amenorrhoea for 6 months and weight gain since she quit smoking. Her urine pregnancy test (UPT) is negative. Her serum hormonal levels are as follows:

Serum estradiol	350 pmol/L
FSH	5 IU/L
LH	15 IU/L

The most likely diagnosis is:

a. Polycystic ovarian disease
b. Premature menopause
c. Endometriosis
d. Ovarian neoplasm
e. Hydatidiform mole

25) Postcoital bleeding may be caused by each of the following EXCEPT:

a. Adenomyosis
b. Atrophic vaginitis
c. Cervical ectropion
d. Cervical polyp
e. Carcinoma of the cervix

26) The most important initial investigation for a sexually active 17-year-old woman complaining of lower abdominal pain and irregular vaginal bleeding is:

a. Transvaginal ultrasonography
b. Urine pregnancy test
c. FBC
d. High vaginal and endometrial swab
e. Serum βhCG and progesterone

27) A 35-year-old woman of 39 weeks' gestation is found to have a fetus in transverse lie presentation confirmed by ultrasonography. The most appropriate management is:

a. Episiotomy
b. Syntocinon i.v.
c. Midforceps rotation
d. Admit and perform external cephalic version (ECV)
e. Hysterectomy

28) A 26-year-old woman complains of dyspareunia. On examination she is found to have a fixed, retroverted uterus and has a tender old laparotomy scar. Treatment for endometriosis may include each of the following EXCEPT:

a. Danazol
b. Norethisterone
c. Total hysterectomy with bilateral salpingo-ophorectomy
d. Diathermy
e. Clomiphene citrate

29) A 19-year-old woman who is a primigravida presents at 22 weeks' gestation. She is noted to have ++ proteinuria and a BP of 170/110. She complains of frontal headache and nausea. You decide to admit her. Appropriate steps in management aside from taking blood include all of the following EXCEPT:

a. 24-hour urine collection for protein
b. Fetal cardiotocogram
c. Consent for emergency caesarean section
d. Transabdominal ultrasonography
e. Intravenous hydralazine or labetalol

30) Appropriate investigations for recurrent miscarriages include the following EXCEPT:

a. Chromosomal karyotyping of both parents
b. Screening for antiphospholipid antibody and lupus anticoagulant
c. Transvaginal ultrasonography
d. Semen analysis
e. Hysterosalpingogram

31) Pelvic inflammatory disease is associated with all of the following EXCEPT:

a. Infertility
b. Ectopic pregnancies
c. *Chlamydia trachomatis* infection
d. Tubo-ovarian abscess
e. Endometriosis

32) A 22-year-old woman presents with frothy grey vaginal discharge. She states that she last had unprotected sexual intercourse 2 weeks ago. The vaginal discharge emits a fishy odour on alkalinization with potassium hydroxide and is noted to have a pH of 5. The most likely organism is:

a. *Neisseria gonorrhoeae*
b. *Trichomonas vaginalis*
c. Candidiasis
d. *Chlamydia trachomatis*
e. *Gardnerella vaginalis*

33) A 50-year-old woman presents with an abdominal mass and back pain. She denies abdominal pain or abnormal vaginal bleeding, having had her last period 9 months ago. Cervical smears have never been abnormal. On examination there is a central mass palpable to above the level of the umbilicus. On pelvic examination there is a palpable right adnexal mass. Urine hCG is negative. The most useful initial investigation is:

a. Plain abdominal and lumbar spine radiographs
b. CT scan of the abdomen and pelvis
c. Serum progesterone and βhCG
d. Pelvic ultrasonography
e. CEA-125 tumour marker

34) A 30-year-old woman who is a primigravida has prolonged labour lasting 18 hours. The cervix is dilated to 8 cm. Fetal monitoring now shows late decelerations and a scalp pH of 7.2. The next course of action is:

a. Episiotomy
b. Syntocinon i.v.
c. Midforceps rotation
d. Vacuum suction delivery
e. Emergency C-section

35) A 20-year-old woman presents with galactorrhoea and amenorrhoea. Her urine pregnancy test is negative. The most likely diagnosis is:

a. Ovarian failure
b. Anorexia
c. Hypothyroidism
d. Prolactinoma
e. Cushing's syndrome

36) A 30-year-old, obese, hirsute woman presents with amenorrhea. Her blood pressure is 170/90 and her urine dipstick is positive for glucose. The most likely diagnosis is:

a. Ovarian failure
b. Anorexia
c. Hypothyroidism
d. Prolactinoma
e. Cushing's syndrome

37) A married, 38-year-old, obese woman of three with varicose veins and a 20 cigarette per day smoking habit would like a form of contraception. The most suitable choice would be:

a. Female condom
b. Contraceptive sponge
c. Combined oral contraceptive
d. Progesterone-only pill
e. Douching

38) A 28-year-old primigravida woman presents with lower abdominal pain and a spiking fever 24 hours after delivery of her baby. The most likely diagnosis is:

a. Mittelschmerz
b. Endometriosis
c. Appendicitis
d. Endometritis
e. Postpartum haemorrhage

39) A 30-year-old multiparous woman presents with scant vaginal bleeding, severe hypotension and a tender uterus. Fetal heart sounds, present previously, are not detected. The most likely diagnosis is:

a. Endometritis
b. Placental abruption
c. Postpartum haemorrhage
d. Placenta praevia
e. Ruptured ectopic pregnancy

40) A 50-year-old woman reports night sweats and hot flushes. What blood test would you order to confirm menopause?

a. FSH
b. LH
c. Progesterone
d. Prolactin
e. Testosterone

41) Candidal infection is associated with the following EXCEPT:

a. Pruritis
b. Glycosuria
c. Increase during pregnancy
d. Immune suppression
e. Is characteristically a frothy yellow–green discharge

42) An increased risk of osteoporosis occurs with the following, EXCEPT:

    a. Heparin
    b. PCOs
    c. Anorexia
    d. Turner's syndrome
    e. Athletic amenorrhoea

43) A 20-year-old primigravida of 36 weeks' gestation presents with a blood pressure of 160/110. What is the next step in management?

    a. Rupture membranes
    b. Emergency C-section
    c. Intravenous Syntocinon
    d. Epidural anaesthesia
    e. Control blood pressure

44) Increased prolactin levels are associated with the following EXCEPT:

    a. Methyldopa
    b. Increased gonadotrophin-releasing hormones
    c. Oligomenorrhoea
    d. Acromegaly
    e. Menorrhagia

45) The following drugs cross the placenta EXCEPT:

    a. Pyrimethamine
    b. Heparin
    c. Warfarin
    d. Tetracycline
    e. Carbimazole

46) A 25-year-old woman with type 1 diabetes mellitus wants to start a family. One of the most important points to discuss is:

    a. Commence a statin
    b. Commence an ACE inhibitor
    c. Start an oral hypoglycaemic drug
    d. Commence folic acid
    e. Reduce dose of insulin

47) Women taking the COC are more susceptible to which ONE of the following:

    a. Ovarian cancer
    b. Cancer of the uterus
    c. Venous thrombosis
    d. Pancreatitis
    e. Benign breast disease

48) Which statement concerning the emergency contraceptive pill is FALSE?

   a. Should be used within 48 hours of unprotected sex
   b. Contains progestogens only
   c. Should be repeated if vomiting occurs
   d. Follow-up should be arranged if there is a delay in the next expected menstrual cycle
   e. Higher doses are required for women with epilepsy

49) The most common malignant tumour that affects women is:

   a. Ovarian cancer
   b. Bowel cancer
   c. Endometrial cancer
   d. Breast cancer
   e. Cervical cancer

50) The most common cause of hirsutism in women is:

   a. Polycystic ovarian syndrome
   b. Idiopathic
   c. Anabolic steroids
   d. Congenital adrenal hyperplasia
   e. Phenytoin

4. Obstetrics and Gynaecology: EMQ Questions

Theme: causes of vaginal discharge

Options

A. *Trichomonas vaginalis*
B. *Gardnerella* spp.
C. *Chlamydia* spp.
D. Gonorrhoea
E. *Mycobacterium tuberculosis*
F. HIV
G. Lymphogranuloma venerum
H. *Treponema pallidum*
I. Granuloma inguinale
J. *Candida albicans*
K. *Staphylococcus aureus*

For each presentation below, choose the SINGLE most likely causative organism from the list of options. Each option may be used once, more than once or not at all.

1) A 22-year-old woman presents with intensely irritating yellowish-green frothy vaginal discharge with severe dyspareunia. The organism is seen best under the microscope in a drop of saline.

2) A 30-year-old pregnant woman presents with a thick, white vaginal discharge associated with irritation of the vulva.

3) A 16-year-old girl who uses tampons presents with cervicitis, urethritis and unilateral Bartholin's gland inflammation.

4) A 28-year-old woman presents with acute, right upper quadrant, abdominal pain and watery vaginal discharge. The organism is detected by microimmunofluorescence.

5) A 23-year-old woman presents with fishy, foul-smelling, vaginal odour. Clue cells are found in the smear.

Theme: treatment of infertility

Options

A. Steroid suppression
B. Laparoscopy
C. Ethinylestradiol from day 1 to day 10
D. Salpingolysis
E. Human menopausal gonadotrophins
F. Clomiphene citrate
G. Ligation of varicocele
H. Intracytoplasmic sperm insemination
I. Artificial insemination with donor semen
J. In vitro fertilization
K. Tubal surgery

For each case below, choose the SINGLE most appropriate treatment from the list of options. Each option may be used once, more than once or not at all.

6) The plasma progesterone level during the luteal phase of the cycle is absent. FSH and LH levels are noted to be low.

7) Agglutination of the sperm head to head is seen on semen analysis. Sperm antibodies are also noted in the man's plasma.

8) The seminal analysis reveals severe oligospermia. The wife has patent tubes and a normal uterus.

9) The postcoital test reveals absence of sperm. The husband has a past history of mumps with orchitis. The wife has patent tubes and a normal uterus.

10) A 35-year-old woman is found to have blocked and severely diseased tubes on laparoscopy and hysterosalpingography. The uterus is normal.

Theme: diagnosis of abdominal pain in pregnancy

Options

A. Peptic ulcer disease
B. Fulminating pre-eclampsia
C. Appendicitis
D. Miscarriage
E. Fibroids
F. Cholecystitis
G. Ectopic pregnancy
H. Urinary infection
I. Ureteric stone
J. Abruptio placentae
K. Hydramnios
L. Pyelonephritis

For each patient below, choose the SINGLE most likely diagnosis from the list of options. Each option may be used once, more than once or not at all.

11) A 33-year-old multiparous woman of 32 weeks' gestation complains of severe back pain. Urinalysis reveals red blood cells. She is apyrexial.

12) A 25-year-old woman who is a primigravida of 8 weeks' gestation presents with severe lower abdominal cramping, vaginal bleeding and the passage of clots. The internal os is open.

13) A 28-year-old woman who is a primigravida of 10 weeks' gestation presents with sudden, severe lower abdominal pain. The abdomen is rigid and the uterus tender.

14) A 30-year-old multiparous woman of 16 weeks' gestation presents with lower abdominal pain and tenderness. On examination she has a fundal height of 25 cm and you palpate a firm mass. She also complains of urinary frequency but denies dysuria. There is only one fetal heart beat.

15) A 26-year-old nulliparous woman of 20 weeks' gestation presents with headache and epigastric pain. BP is 150/100 and rising.

Theme: causes of genital tract bleeding in early pregnancy

Options

A. Inevitable miscarriage
B. Missed miscarriage
C. Complete miscarriage
D. Threatened miscarriage
E. Incomplete miscarriage
F. Hydatidiform mole
G. Recurrent miscarriage
H. Cervical polyp
I. Cancer of the cervix
J. Ectopic pregnancy
K. Cervical erosion

For each case below, choose the SINGLE most likely cause from the list of options. Each option may be used once, more than once or not at all.

16) A nulliparous woman of 10 weeks' gestation presents with per vagina bleeding and pain. The internal os is open. There has been no passage of products of conception.

17) A woman who is a primigravida of 8 weeks' gestation presents with painless per vagina bleeding. Serum and urinary hCG levels are much higher than expected for her gestation.

18) A woman who is a primigravida of 20 weeks' gestation has a small uterus that is not consistent with her last menstrual period date. She has had no per vagina bleeding. She has not felt the baby move all week and there are no fetal heart sounds on ultrasonography.

19) A multiparous woman of 9 weeks' gestation presents with per vagina bleeding. The internal os is not dilated. The cervix is normal.

20) A primiparous woman of 10 weeks' gestation presents with per vagina bleeding and passage of products of conception. The cervical os remains open.

Theme: pelvic masses

Options

A. Endometriosis
B. Dermoid cyst
C. Ovarian carcinoma
D. Tubo-ovarian abscess
E. Pelvic inflammatory disease
F. Endometrial carcinoma
G. Ectopic pregnancy
H. Urinary tract infection

For each case below, choose the SINGLE most likely cause from the list of options. Each option may be used once, more than once or not at all.

21) A 55-year-old woman presents with a lower abdominal mass. The mass is palpated in the left iliac fossa. An ultrasound scan shows a mass with solid and cystic echogenicity and fluid in the pouch of Douglas.

22) A 30-year-old pregnant woman has her routine 18-week ultrasound scan. The scan shows a mass with complex solid and cystic echogenic patterns.

23) A 35-year-old woman presents with a longstanding history of dysmenorrhoea. On examination there is tenderness in the pouch of Douglas. Ultrasound scan shows a cystic lesion with numerous echogenic substances.

24) A 45-year-old, monogamous, sexually active woman presents with dysuria, frequency and haematuria. There is no history of vaginal discharge.

25) A 35-year-old woman is being treated for PID and seems to be recovering well. After a few days she develops a high temperature. Ultrasound scan shows a cystic mass.

4. Obstetrics and Gynaecology: SBA/BOF Answers

1) b.
Guidelines for anti-D immunoglobulin suggest prophylaxis under the following sensitizing circumstances: spontaneous miscarriage after 12 weeks' gestation; spontaneous miscarriage with instrumentation (termination of pregnancy or TOP); threatened miscarriage at any gestation, after falls or abdominal trauma. The dose of anti-D immunoglobulin is determined according to the level of exposure to rhesus-positive blood. Anti-D should be offered within 72 hours and covers the mother for the next 6 weeks. Anti-D prophylaxis is repeated at this time if bleeding persists. Routine antenatal prophylaxis according to The Royal College of Obstetricians and Gynaecologists for all rhesus-negative women consists of two doses of at least 500 IU anti-D immunoglobulin, the first dose at 28 weeks' gestation and the second at 34 weeks' gestation.

2) c.
Risk factors for endometrial cancer include nulliparity, late menopause, diabetes, history of unopposed oestrogen administration, oestrogen-secreting tumours of the ovaries and obesity. Premarin is a form of unopposed oestrogen HRT and should be administered to women only post-hysterectomy.

3) e.
Routine blood tests offered at booking clinic include full blood count, blood group and antibody screen, serology for hepatitis B (not A!), syphilis, rubella and HIV. Sickle cell test and haemoglobin electrophoresis are also offered to at-risk patients.

4) d.
Increased levels of human chorionic gonadotrophin (hCG) have been associated with choriocarcinoma, hyperemesis gravidarum, pregnancy and hydatidiform mole. Hepatoma may be associated with increased levels of α-fetoprotein. Ovarian cancer may be associated with elevated CA-125.

5) a.
Cervical smear may pick up incidental infections such as *Trichomonas vaginalis*, bacterial vaginosis (*Gardnerella* sp.), and *Actinomyces* and *Candida* spp. Cervical smear may reveal mild-to-severe dysplasia which is suggestive of low- to high-grade CIN (cervical invasive neoplasia). Severe dyskaryosis with additional features may suggest invasive carcinoma.

Dyskaryotic glandular cells may represent adenocarcinoma of the endometrium or endocervical adenocarcinoma *in situ*.

6) e.
The Mirena coil or the levonorgestrel-releasing intrauterine system (IUS) is licensed to be used for 5 years at a time in the UK. It has a product licence for control of menorrhagia. The local effect of the Mirena coil causes thickening of the cervical mucus, endometrial atrophy and partial ovulation suppression. It is not advisable in patients with a past history of PID and does not increase the risk of ectopic pregnancy. By acting as a contraceptive device with 99% efficacy, the risk is lower.

7) e.
Postcoital bleeding is associated with cervical polyp, cervical ectropion, carcinoma of the cervix, infection with *Trichomonas vaginalis*, which may appear as a strawberry cervix, and atrophic vaginitis.

8) d.
Deep dyspareunia is associated with PID, endometriosis, ectopic pregnancy, ovarian neoplasm and chronic pelvic pain. Superficial dyspareunia is associated with vulvar, vaginal or urethral pathology.

9) a.
Intermenstrual bleeding may be associated with infection in patients with an IUCD *in situ* and with intramural or submucous fibroids.

10) d.
The differential diagnosis in this situation includes endometritis, retained products of conception, haematoma and breakdown of sutures.

11) d.
Other causes for preterm labour include procedures such as amniocentesis, multiple pregnancy and an abnormal uterus.

12) e.
Other potential complications of pre-eclampsia include fits, disseminated intravascular coagulopathy (DIC) and maternal death.

13) a.
Dianette oral contraceptive pill contains the antiandrogen cytoproterone acetate.

14) d.
Causes of dysmenorrhoea include endometriosis, misplaced IUCD, pelvic inflammatory disease, ovarian tumour, history of sexual abuse, and prior abdominal or pelvic surgery. Fibroids are associated with menorrhagia. Polycystic ovaries are associated with amenorrhoea.

15) d.

An ectopic pregnancy is a pregnancy that occurs outside the uterine cavity. The majority occur in the fallopian tube. Isthmal pregnancies may rupture between 4 and 8 weeks because the wall of the medial two-thirds of the tube cannot stretch. Ampullary pregnancies may rupture between 8 and 12 weeks, as the muscle wall of the lateral third of the tube is lax. It occurs in 1 in 200 pregnancies and is associated with salpingitis, tubal surgery, IUCD, etc. It may present with shoulder-tip pain due to diaphragmatic irritation from accumulated blood. The abdominal pain may be bilateral or unilateral. Classically, the patient will have sudden, severe, lower quadrant abdominal pain, a rigid abdomen, a very tender uterus and a boggy adnexal mass.

16) e.

The combined oral contraceptive pill contains oestrogen, which is absorbed in breast milk and therefore should not be offered as postpartum contraception.

17) b.

The differential diagnosis for postmenopausal bleeding includes carcinoma of the cervix and endometrium, endometrial polyp and atrophic vaginitis. A speculum examination of the cervix and a cervical smear are indicated. An urgent transvaginal ultrasound scan should be arranged to assess for endometrial hyperplasia or the presence of a polyp. A pipelle biopsy of the endometrium can then be taken if the endometrium is thickened.

18) b.

This is an NSAID that reduces contractions of the uterus by inhibiting prostaglandin synthesis.

19) e.

Zoladex is a GnRH (gonadotrophin-releasing hormone) agonist.

20) b.

Emergency contraception in the form of Levonelle may be offered up to 72 hours after unprotected sexual intercourse. The IUCD may be offered up to 5 days after unprotected sexual intercourse. The Mirena coil is not recommended for emergency contraception.

21) a.

The patient should be type and cross-matched for 6 units of blood.

22) b.

23) b.
Endometriosis is a condition in which the cells of the inner lining of the uterus, the endometrium, are deposited outside the uterine cavity. Up to 30% of women undergoing investigations for infertility have been found to have endometriosis at laparoscopy.

24) a.
PCOS is associated with a serum LH:FSH ratio of 3. Diagnosis is confirmed by transvaginal ultrasonography that will demonstrate the typical follicles surrounding the ovary.

25) a.
Postcoital bleeding may be caused by atrophic vaginitis, cervical ectropion, cervical carcinoma or cervical polyp. Cervical ectropion is eversion of the lower cervical canal and is associated with the three 'Ps' – puberty, pregnancy and the combined oral contraceptive pill. It is usually asymptomatic but can present with postcoital bleeding. Treatment involves cryotherapy.

26) b.
The diagnosis of ectopic pregnancy should be excluded.

27) d.
ECV involves externally rotating the baby from a breech or transverse lie to cephalic. Complications may include placental abruption and premature rupture of membranes so the manoeuvre is carried out in hospital in case an emergency caesarean section is required.

28) e.
Clomiphene citrate is used to induce ovulation.

29) c.
This patient has pre-eclampsia. As this patient is only 22 weeks pregnant, management is tailored to prolonging pregnancy subject to continuous fetal and maternal monitoring. In later stages of pregnancy or in severe pre-eclampsia delivery is required.

30) d.
Causes for recurrent miscarriages include SLE, antiphospholipid syndrome, endocrine disorders (diabetes, PCOS), thrombophilias, anatomical variations and chromosomal disorders.

31) e.

32) e.
This is the most common vaginal infection in women of child-bearing age. Treatment is with a course of metronidazole.

33) d.

The mass is an ovarian tumour. Over 90% of these carcinomas originate from ovarian epithelial cells. Ovarian cancer is the most common gynaecological malignancy.

34) e.

The late deceleration and low pH suggest that the baby is in distress and an emergency C-section is required.

35) d.

Other symptoms include headaches, visual disturbances and infertility. Prolactinomas are associated with prolactin levels of at least 2000 mU/L.

36) e.

Cushing's syndrome is caused by abnormally high levels of cortisol. In a large proportion of patients the high levels of cortisol are caused by a pituitary adenoma producing high levels of ACTH (Cushing's disease).

37) d.

The COC is contraindicated in this patient and as the other forms of contraception have low efficacy rates the POP is the most suitable choice.

38) d.

Endometritis occurs when microorganisms harboured in the vaginal canal ascend to infect the endometrium. Commonly isolated organisms include group B streptococci, enterococci and staphylococci. Risk factors include caesarean section, prolonged rupture of membranes, retained products of conception and instrumental delivery.

39) b.

40) a.

An FSH level >30 IU/L with amenorrhoea is diagnostic of the menopause. In the UK the average age of the menopause is 51.

41) e.

A frothy yellow–green discharge is associated with *Trichomonas vaginalis*.

42) b.

43) e.

The patient should be admitted for close monitoring and further investigations.

44) b.

45) b.
Pyrimethamine is an antimalarial and is a folate inhibitor. Warfarin is a known teratogen, Tetracyclines cross the placenta and accumulate in fetal bones, causing impaired development and can also cause cosmetic staining of teeth. Carbimazole can cause hypothyroidism in the fetus.

46) d.
Women with diabetes mellitus are at high risk of conceiving a child with a neural tube defect. Other high-risk groups include women with coeliac disease, sickle cell anaemia, women taking antiepileptic medication and those who have had a previous pregnancy with a neural tube defect. High-risk groups should take 5 mg folate daily (as opposed to 400 μg) until week 12 of pregnancy.

47) c.
The COC predisposes to the formation of thrombosis by increasing the levels of a number of coagulation factors (e.g. factor VII) and by reducing the levels of several coagulation inhibitors (e.g. antithrombin, and proteins C and S).

48) a.
The emergency contraceptive pill can be used within 72 hours of unprotected sex.

49) d.
After breast cancer, colorectal and then lung cancer are the most common cancers in women.

50) b.

4. Obstetrics and Gynaecology: EMQ Answers

1) A.
TV is a sexually transmitted infection (STI). It is a motile flagellate protozoa, which thrives under conditions that raise the vaginal pH >5.0. Speculum examination will show a typical strawberry appearance due to microscopic haemorrhages.

2) J.
This is a yeast that proliferates under conditions when the vaginal pH is more alkaline. Risk factors include pregnancy, immunocompromised women, diabetes mellitus and broad-spectrum antibiotics.

3) D.
Neissseria gonorrhoeae is sexually transmitted and is an intracellular aerobic diplococcus. In the UK it is the second most common STI, the most common being chlamydia infection.

4) C.
The patient has Fitz–Hugh–Curtis syndrome, which occurs as a complication to pelvic inflammatory disease. Ascending pelvic infection results in inflammation of the liver capsule and formation of perihepatic adhesions. This syndrome can be caused by *Chlamydia* spp. or gonorrhoea. The ELISA (enzyme-linked immunosorbent assay) test detects chlamydia antigens.

5) B.
Clue cells are found on microscopy and are actually vaginal epithelial cells that have bacteria attached to the cells' surface, giving a serrated appearance.

6) F.
The absent progesterone levels suggests that ovulation is not occurring. Clomiphene citrate causes inhibition of oestrogen feedback on the hypothalamus and therefore stimulates release of FSH and LH from the pituitary, causing follicular growth and ovulation.

7) A.
Injury or infection of the testes can cause production of antibodies against sperm, which leads to agglutination and therefore motility disorders.

8) H.

9) I.

10) J.

11) I.
Ureteric stones occur I in 2000 pregnancies and usually in the second and third trimesters.

12) D.

13) G.
An ectopic pregnancy may manifest between the fourth and tenth weeks of gestation. This patient needs emergency surgery to stem the bleeding from a ruptured fallopian tube.

14) E.
Central necrosis (red degeneration) is one of the complications of fibroids and is seen in pregnancy. Degeneration occurs when the fibroid enlarges during pregnancy, causing it to outgrow its blood supply.

15) B.

16) A.
The os is open therefore miscarriage is inevitable.

17) F.
In normal pregnancies levels of hCG should double every 48 hours. Higher than expected hCG levels may indicate a multiple pregnancy, molar pregnancy or a miscalculated date of conception.

18) B.
In a missed miscarriage the os will be closed and the uterus smaller than expected. Symptoms of pregnancy such as tender breasts, nausea and fatigue may also diminish.

19) D.

20) E.

21) C.

Echogenicity relates to the ability of a tissue to reflect back sound waves, also known as echoes. Ovarian carcinomas are mostly epithelial in origin and have a variable proportion of solid and cystic components.

22) B.

Solid components of a dermoid cyst may contain mature tissue such as hair and teeth.

23) A.

24) H.

25) D.

5. PAEDIATRICS

In these questions candidates must select one answer only.

1) A 7-year-old boy presents with an itchy anus. His mother states that the itching is worse at night in bed. The most likely diagnosis is:

   a. Enterobiasis
   b. Ascariasis
   c. Scabies
   d. Body lice
   e. Crab lice

2) Treatment for this boy would be:

   a. Derbac-M
   b. Malathion
   c. Mebendazole
   d. Pyrantel pamoate
   e. Permethrin

3) A 10-year-old boy presents with allergic nasal polyps. What is the best treatment for this boy?

   a. Betnesol nasal drops
   b. Clarityn
   c. Zirtek
   d. Saline nasal drops
   e. Xylometazoline nasal drops

4) A 4-year-old boy presents with fever, epistaxis and pain in his legs. On examination he has hepatosplenomegaly. The most useful blood test is:

   a. LFTs
   b. FBC
   c. U&Es
   d. ESR
   e. Creatine kinase

5) A 15-year-old girl presents with fever and sore throat. On examination there is an exudate over both tonsils. She has no drug allergies. The most appropriate treatment is:

   a. Amoxicillin
   b. Penicillin
   c. Metronidazole
   d. Ciprofloxacin
   e. Co-amoxiclavulanic acid

6) A 5-year-old boy presents with a maculopapular rash on his buttocks and ankles. He also complains of abdominal pain and knee pain. The most likely diagnosis is:

   a. Rheumatic fever
   b. Juvenile chronic arthritis
   c. Coeliac disease
   d. Henoch–Schönlein syndrome
   e. Chickenpox

7) A 4-year-old girl presents with pallor, irritability, abdominal distension and fatty diarrhoea. Full blood count shows both a macrocytic and a microcytic anaemia. The next most useful investigation is:

   a. Sweat sodium and chloride test
   b. Abdominal radiograph
   c. Hydrogen breath test
   d. Endomysial antibody
   e. Abdominal ultrasonography

8) A 6-week-old baby boy is brought in by his mother for failure to thrive. He vomits his food across the room after each feed. His mother states that he is always hungry. The most useful investigation is:

   a. Test feed
   b. Contrast enema
   c. Ultrasonography
   d. Abdominal radiograph
   e. Sweat chloride test

9) Treatment would be:

   a. Oral rehydration therapy
   b. Ramstedt's operation
   c. Reduction with contrast enema
   d. Gluten-free diet
   e. Pancreatic enzyme supplementation

10) An 18-month-old baby presents with fever and vomiting. The throat, chest and abdomen are normal on examination. The most likely diagnosis is:

   a. Gastroenteritis
   b. Viral meningitis
   c. Pharyngeal pouch
   d. Intussusception
   e. Congenital hiatal hernia

11) An 8-year-old girl presents with fever, drowsiness and a non-blanching rash. The most likely diagnosis is:

   a. Infectious mononucleosis
   b. Meningitis
   c. Scarlet fever
   d. Chickenpox
   e. Kawasaki's syndrome

12) The most useful investigation is:

   a. FBC
   b. Blood cultures
   c. Lumbar puncture
   d. Monospot test
   e. Throat swab

13) The most appropriate treatment is:

   a. Benzylpenicillin
   b. Erythromycin
   c. Aspirin
   d. Chloramphenicol
   e. Cefuroxime

14) Dietary iron is required by the age of:

   a. 2 months
   b. 4 months
   c. 6 months
   d. 10 months
   e. 12 months

15) An 18-month-old boy presents with fever, bleeding from the lips and an erythematous rash over the face and trunk. The boy does not like to hold anything in his hands and refuses to stand up. The most likely diagnosis is:

   a. Streptococcal scarlet fever
   b. Leptospirosis
   c. Epstein–Barr viral infection
   d. Erythema multiforme
   e. Kawasaki's syndrome

16) The most appropriate management would be:

   a. Admit the boy to hospital and give daily aspirin
   b. Admit the boy to hospital for intravenous penicillin
   c. Admit the boy to hospital for intravenous corticosteroids
   d. Treat as an outpatient with oral penicillin
   e. Treat at home symptomatically with Calpol (paracetamol) as needed

17) A 4-month-old baby is brought in by his mother. She states that he had been coughing for a few days and is now wheezing and breathless. On examination the baby is febrile with a temperature of 38°C and is breathing at a rate of 70/min with intercostal recession. Widespread râles and rhonchi are present on auscultation of the chest. The most likely diagnosis is:

a. Asthma
b. Pneumonia
c. Bronchiolitis
d. Whooping cough
e. Acute laryngotracheitis

18) A 7-year-old boy presents with fever, vomiting and abdominal pain. On examination he is tender in the periumbilical region and in the right lower abdomen. He looks pale and has no appetite. The most likely diagnosis is:

a. Intussusception
b. Gastroenteritis
c. Cystic fibrosis
d. Appendicitis
e. Ulcerative colitis

19) A 14-year-old girl presents with vomiting and severe abdominal pain. She states that she had a sore throat a week ago. This afternoon, she had been playing rugby at school and been knocked in her side. On examination she is pale, apyrexial and acutely tender in the left upper abdomen. The most likely diagnosis is:

a. Splenic rupture
b. Hepatic rupture
c. Acute appendicitis
d. Perforated peptic ulcer
e. Acute intestinal obstruction

20) For which condition is the pneumococcal vaccine indicated over the age of 2?

a. Cerebral palsy
b. Coeliac disease
c. Sickle cell trait
d. Diabetes insipidus
e. Cystic fibrosis

21) A 4-year-old girl is brought in by her mother. The mother states that her daughter has nightmares and snores. She has a history of recurrent ear infections. On examination the child has large tonsils and nasal speech. The most likely diagnosis is:

a. Adenoidal hyperplasia
b. Sleep apnoea
c. Asthma
d. Nasal polyps
e. Gastro-oesophageal reflux disease

22) A 12-year-old girl presents with a pink macular truncal rash and suboccipital lymphadenopathy. The most likely diagnosis is:

a. Mumps
b. Chickenpox
c. Rubella
d. Measles
e. Erythema infectiosum

23) A 2-year-old girl is able to do the following EXCEPT:

a. Use two to three words in a sentence
b. Turn pages of a book
c. Follow a two-step command
d. Participate in group play
e. Turn a door knob

24) A 6-year-old girl presents with fever and vesicles on the palms and soles and in the mouth. She is drooling saliva and is very irritable. The most likely aetiology is:

a. Coxsackie A16 virus infection
b. Herpes simplex virus infection
c. Human parvovirus type B12
d. *Treponema pallidum*
e. Measles

25) A 15-year-old presents with an oval pink rash. She states that it started with a single patch that became scaly but has now spread all over her chest. The most likely diagnosis is:

a. Scarlet fever
b. Pityriasis rosea
c. Rubella
d. Psoriasis
e. Discoid eczema

26) A 6-month-old baby is brought in with a nappy rash. On examination the rash is isolated red plaques and covered with silvery scales. The most likely diagnosis is:

a. Ammonia dermatitis
b. Seborrhoeic eczema dermatitis
c. Candida dermatitis
d. Psoriatic dermatitis
e. Cellulitis

27) The following are recognized causes of short stature EXCEPT for:

a. Achondroplasia
b. Coeliac disease
c. Hypopituitarism
d. Homocystinuria
e. Constitutional

28) An 8-year-old girl presents with epistaxis and knee pain. On examination she is pale, tachycardic and apyrexial. A pansystolic murmur is auscultated. She has a serpiginous, red, raised rash over her trunk and non-tender subcutaneous nodules near her joints. The most likely diagnosis is:

a. Idiopathic thrombocytopenic purpura
b. Juvenile rheumatoid arthritis
c. Kawasaki's disease
d. Rubella
e. Rheumatic fever

29) The following investigations are indicated EXCEPT:

a. A 12-lead ECG
b. FBC
c. ESR
d. Antistreptolysin O test
e. Creatine kinase

30) The most appropriate treatment is:

a. Aspirin
b. Benzylpenicillin
c. Corticosteroid therapy
d. NSAIDs
e. Cefuroxime

31) A 5-month-old baby boy is brought in by his mother. She states that he has blood and mucus in his stool. He had recently been changed from milk to solids. He has episodes of screaming and abdominal pain but appears well between attacks. The most likely diagnosis is:

   a. Volvulus
   b. Intussusception
   c. Gastroenteritis
   d. Anal fissure
   e. Meckel's diverticulum

32) A 13-year-old boy presents with fever, sore throat and right hip pain. You suspect irritable hip. Appropriate investigations include all of the following EXCEPT:

   a. FBC
   b. ESR
   c. Ultrasonography of the hip
   d. Radiograph of the hip
   e. Bone scan

33) Appropriate management includes all of the following EXCEPT:

   a. High-dose regular paracetamol
   b. Skin traction
   c. Skeletal traction
   d. Bed rest
   e. 24-hour observation for repeated temperature checks

34) What is the electrolyte imbalance associated with pyloric stenosis?

   a. Hyperchloraemic alkalosis
   b. Hypochloraemic alkalosis
   c. Hyponatraemia
   d. Hyperkalaemia
   e. Metabolic acidosis

35) Koplik's spots are seen in the following condition:

   a. Measles
   b. Mumps
   c. Rubella
   d. Scarlet fever
   e. Erythema infectiosum

36) A 4-year old boy presents with anorexia, nausea and vomiting. On examination, he has a blue line on the gums and is noted to have a foot drop. A blood test reveals anaemia. The most likely cause of poisoning is:

   a. Lead
   b. Paracetamol
   c. Methanol
   d. Cyanide
   e. Mercury

37) A 4-year-old child presents to A&E with a high fever and stridorous breathing. He is sitting forward and drooling saliva. He requires intubation for respiratory distress. The most appropriate antibiotic treatment is:

   a. Amoxicillin
   b. Vancomycin
   c. Trimethoprim
   d. Cefotaxime
   e. Tetracycline

38) A 12-year-old girl presents with pallor, dyspnoea and a pulse rate of 190. She is noted to have cardiomegaly and hepatomegaly. The most likely diagnosis is:

   a. Kawasaki's disease
   b. Mitral stenosis
   c. Congestive heart failure
   d. Congenital nephrotic syndrome
   e. Myocarditis

39) A 10-year-old boy presents to A&E after fainting during gym. On examination, he has a loud systolic ejection murmur with a thrill. The most likely diagnosis is:

   a. Mitral stenosis
   b. Aortic stenosis
   c. Pericarditis
   d. Congestive heart failure
   e. Myocarditis

40) A 12-year-old boy presents to A&E with a red, painful, swollen scrotum. His MSU is normal. The most likely diagnosis is:

   a. Ureteric colic
   b. Testicular tumour
   c. Hydrocele
   d. Testicular torsion
   e. Phimosis

41) A 3-year-old boy presents with a 3-day history of noisy breathing on inspiration and a barking cough worse at night. He has a low-grade fever and is hoarse. The most likely diagnosis is:

a. Influenza
b. Asthma
c. Croup
d. Pneumonia
e. Allergic rhinitis

42) A 4-year-old presents to the GP for night terrors and loud snoring. On examination he is a mouth breather and has large tonsils that meet at the midline. The most likely cause is:

a. Asthma
b. Retrotonsillar abscess
c. Obstructive sleep apnoea
d. Sinusitis
e. Gastro-oesophageal reflux disease

43) A 10-year-old thin boy presents with chronic cough. A chest radiograph reveals bronchiectasis. He also has steatorrhoea. The most likely diagnosis is:

a. Asthma
b. Coeliac disease
c. Cystic fibrosis
d. Chest infection
e. Croup

44) A 4-year-old boy presents with bone pain and weakness. Investigations reveal a pancytopenia and blasts. The most likely diagnosis is:

a. Acute lymphoblastic leukaemia
b. Multiple myeloma
c. Acute myeloid leukaemia
d. Chronic lymphocytic leukaemia
e. Chronic myeloid leukaemia

45) A 10-year-old boy presents with a boiled sweet stuck in his throat. He is in respiratory distress and cyanotic. The most appropriate initial management is:

a. Heimlich's manoeuvre
b. Intramuscular adrenaline 1:1000
c. Endotracheal intubation
d. Tracheostomy
e. Intravenous dexamethasone

46) The Guthrie test is carried out for the screening of which condition:
   a. Phenylketonuria
   b. Congenital hypothyroidism
   c. Cystic fibrosis
   d. MCAD (medium-chain acyl-CoA dehydrogenase) deficiency
   e. Sickle cell disease

47) The Guthrie test should be carried out at what age:
   a. 4 months
   b. 3 months
   c. 2 months
   d. 14 days
   e. 7 days

48) A 13-year-old boy with a BMI of 29 has pain in his thigh and knee and is limping. Movements at the hip are limited. The most likely diagnosis is:
   a. Growing pains
   b. Perthes' disease
   c. Slipped upper femoral epiphysis
   d. Transient synovitis of the hip
   e. Fractured femur

49) A 9-year-old boy presents with a 2-day history of a sore throat and fever. He has now developed a truncal rash and has a strawberry tongue. The most likely diagnosis is:
   a. Measles
   b. Scarlet fever
   c. Chickenpox
   d. Mumps
   e. Rubella

50) Coronary artery aneurysms are associated with the following condition:
   a. Meningitis
   b. Kawasaki's disease
   c. Hand, foot and mouth disease
   d. Henoch–Schönlein disease
   e. Pneumonia

5. Paediatrics: EMQ Questions

Theme: diagnosis of childhood illnesses

Options

A. Measles
B. Rubella
C. Varicella-zoster
D. Mumps
E. Erythema infectiosum
F. Infectious mononucleosis
G. Tuberculosis
H. Typhus
I. Kawasaki's syndrome
J. Pneumococcal meningitis
K. *Haemophilus influenzae* epiglottitis
L. Streptococcal throat infection

For each patient below, choose the SINGLE most likely diagnosis from the list of options. Each option may be used once, more than once or not at all.

1) A 15-year-old girl presents with fever, cough, coryza and conjunctivitis 9 days after exposure. On examination, she has blue–white punctate lesions on the buccal mucosa.

2) A 17-year-old boy presents with fever, stridor and trismus. He is noted to be drooling saliva. On examination he has palpable neck nodes. He fails to respond to a course of penicillin.

3) A 7-year-old girl presents with a low-grade fever and a 'slapped-cheek', erythematous eruption on her cheeks.

4) A 4-year-old boy presents with an acute onset of fever and a vesicular eruption, following an incubation period of 12 days. The vesicles evolve into pustules and crust over.

5) A 1-year-old baby boy presents with a 5-day history of fever, strawberry tongue and erythema of the palms and soles. He also has an enlarged 2-cm lymph node.

Theme: investigation of failure to thrive

Options
A. FBC
B. Sweat test
C. Urinalysis
D. Serum electrolytes
E. Bone films
F. TFTs
G. Buccal smear (girls)
H. Stool culture
I. Echocardiogram
J. Fasting blood glucose
K. Abdominal ultrasonography

For each presentation below, choose the SINGLE most discriminating investigation from the list of options. Each option may be used once, more than once or not at all.

6) A small 6-year-old boy on regular salbutamol inhaler presents with nasal obstruction and persistent cough. On examination he is found to have nasal polyps.

7) A 2-year-old boy presents with anorexia, impaired growth, abdominal distension, abnormal stools and hypotonia. He is irritable when examined.

8) A 14-year-old girl presents with anorexia. She reports that her appetite is good but she cannot seem to gain weight. Her parents describe her as hyperactive and emotional. Blood pressure is 130/80 and pulse rate 108/min.

9) A 5-year-old boy presents with weight loss and nocturnal enuresis. His parents describe him as having profound mood swings. They have attempted to limit his fluid intake at night.

10) A 6-week-old baby presents with failure to thrive. The mother reports that he takes 1 hour for feeding with frequent rests. On examination he is tachycardic, tachypnoeic and has an enlarged liver.

Theme: investigations of paediatric emergencies

Options

A. FBC
B. Serum glucose
C. Skull radiograph
D. Chest radiograph
E. Urinalysis
F. ESR
G. Serum U&Es
H. CT scan of the head
I. Lateral soft-tissue neck radiograph

For each case below, choose the SINGLE most discriminating investigation from the list of options. Each option may be used once, more than once or not at all.

11) An 8-month-old baby is brought to A&E by her mother after falling off the sofa on to her head. On examination she is irritable and alert, with no lateralizing signs. There is a haematoma over her left occiput.

12) A 6-year-old girl is brought to A&E by her mother after falling off a climbing frame in the school playground. On examination there is no deformity or swelling of her extremities. Instead she has bruising of various colours over her arms and tender ribs on palpation.

13) A 2-year-old girl is brought to A&E by her father after falling down the stairs. She is drowsy and has vomited twice. On examination there is a swelling over her occiput. Her pupils are sluggish to respond. Blood pressure is 120/70 and pulse rate is 60.

14) A 2-year-old boy has swallowed a 50 pence coin and points to his throat. He is not distressed.

15) A 4-year-old girl is brought to A&E with severe left shoulder and left upper abdominal pain. Temperature is 40°C. Breath sounds are decreased in the left lung base. Urine dipstick shows scant red blood cells.

Theme: management of paediatric gastrointestinal disorders

Options

A. Vancomycin
B. Panproctocolectomy
C. Gluten-free diet
D. Pancreatic enzyme supplementation
E. Barium enema
F. Rectal biopsy
G. D-Penicillamine and avoidance of chocolates, nuts and shellfish
H. Diverting colostomy
I. Loperamide

For each case below, choose the SINGLE most appropriate management option from the list of options. Each option may be used once, more than once or not at all.

16) A 2-year-old girl presents with failure to thrive and diarrhoea. She is found to have iron-deficiency anaemia. Small bowel biopsy shows flattened villi, elongated crypts and loss of columnar cells.

17) A 12-year-old boy is being treated for osteomyelitis. He has been on intravenous antibiotics for 2 weeks. He now has diarrhoea. On sigmoidoscopy there are multiple, patchy, yellowish areas of necrotic mucosa.

18) A 6-month-old baby boy presents with repeated bouts of vomiting and abdominal distension. He is normal between attacks. A sausage-shaped mass is palpated in his abdomen.

19) A 2-month-old baby girl presents with failure to thrive. She has frequent episodes of vomiting with abdominal distension. Abdominal radiograph shows proximal bowel dilatation and no faeces or gas in the rectum.

20) A 12-year-old boy presents with liver disease. A slit-lamp examination reveals Kayser–Fleischer rings in his cornea. Urinary copper level is high.

Theme: paediatric pathology

Options

A. Surfactant deficiency
B. α_1-Antitrypsin deficiency
C. Hepatic enzyme deficiency
D. Chloride channel defect
E. Allergy
F. Immune defect
G. Viral titre

For each case below, choose the SINGLE most appropriate management option from the list of options. Each option may be used once, more than once or not at all.

21) A baby is born prematurely at 30 weeks' gestation and is having breathing difficulties.

22) A screening test carried out on a 1-week-old baby for cystic fibrosis comes back positive.

23) A 6-month-old baby is diagnosed with an acute case of bronchiolitis.

24) A 30-year-old woman has a past history of recurrent jaundice as a child; she has recently been diagnosed with emphysema.

25) A screening test carried out on a 1-week-old baby for phenylketonuria comes back positive.

5. Paediatrics: SBA/BOF Answers

1) a.
Also known as threadworms, enterobiasis is particularly common in children. The female lays eggs at night, therefore causing intense itching. Ingestion or inhalation of eggs causes infection of the intestines, which manifests as anal pruritis or very occasionally abdominal pain.

2) c.
This should be prescribed to all household members. Strict hygiene measures are also indicated.

3) a.
Betnesol contains betamethasone, a corticosteroid, and helps reduce inflammation.

4) b.
The patient's diagnosis is most probably acute lymphoblastic leukaemia, which can be confirmed on bone marrow biopsy.

5) b.
A fever and exudative tonsillitis can be seen in group A streptococcal pharyngitis and infectious mononucleosis. As only lab tests (swabs/blood test) can differentiate between viral and bacterial aetiology, empirical treatment of this patient should start with penicillin. Amoxicillin should never be prescribed for sore throat as the patient may have infectious mononucleosis and develop a drug rash.

6) d.
This is an autoimmune vasculitis (IgA mediated) mostly seen in children. It usually follows an upper respiratory tract infection (URTI).

7) d.
Endomysial antibody suggests coeliac disease. Definitive diagnosis is made by jejunal biopsy.

8) a.
On test feed, an olive-shaped mass may be palpated and visible peristalsis evident in pyloric stenosis.

9) b.
This involves dissecting the thickened pylorus to widen the gastric outlet.

10) a.

11) b.

12) c.
This will confirm the diagnosis. The CSF obtained will show typical changes, e.g. high number of polymorphs, low glucose levels, high protein levels and a turbid appearance of the fluid.

13) a.
Intramuscular or intravenous benzylpenicillin should be given immediately.

14) c.
Iron stores start to deplete at 6 months of age; exclusive milk feeding does not contain adequate amounts of iron for this stage of growth, so the introduction of solid foods is recommended.

15) e.
The boy will refuse his toys and refuse to stand as the palms and soles will be red and indurated.

16) a.
There is a risk of coronary artery aneurysm associated with Kawasaki's disease.

17) c.

18) d.
McBurney's point lies in the right iliac fossa. The point is one-third the distance between the anterior superior iliac spine (ASIS) and umbilicus.

19) a.
The girl most probably had infectious mononucleosis, which carries a risk of splenic rupture, and contact sports should be avoided for up to 6 weeks post-infection.

20) b.
Other conditions include diabetes mellitus, sickle cell anaemia and asplenia.

21) a.
Adenoidal hyperplasia may present with night terrors, adenoid facies, eustachian tube dysfunction and snoring. Adenoidal hyperplasia can co-exist with enlarged tonsils.

22) c.

23) d.
At this age toddlers will play alongside other children (parallel play) as opposed to playing together.

24) a.
This child has hand, foot and mouth disease.

25) b.
Pityriasis rosea is a self-limiting viral illness associated with Herald's patch.

26) d.

27) d.
Homocystinuria is associated with tall stature.

28) e.
Fever is not always present in cases of acute rheumatic fever, so do not be misled.

29) e.
Rheumatic fever remains a major cause of death and heart disorders in developing countries. It is a systemic condition caused by an untreated infection with group A streptococci.

30) b.

31) b.
Intussusception occurs when a bowel segment telescopes into another segment of bowel. On abdominal palpation this can be felt as a sausage-like mass.

32) e.
Ultrasonography is useful to exclude effusion of the hip or septic arthritis.

33) c.
Daily temperature checks are necessary to rule out septic arthritis.

34) b.

35) a.
These are red spots with white centres seen on the oral mucosa during the early phase of measles.

36) a.
Lead poisoning can occur from consumption of lead-based paint chips or contaminated water from lead-based pipes. Lead lines can be seen at the metaphysis of growing bones on a radiograph.

37) d.
Cefotaxime is the drug of choice for *Haemophilus influenzae* epiglottitis.

38) c.

39) b.

40) d.
This is a urological emergency. The spermatic cord, which contains the testicular artery, twists, resulting in a diminished blood supply to the testis and testicular necrosis.

41) c.
Croup is often preceded by a mild URTI and is usually caused by the parainfluenza virus.

42) c.
Causes of obstructive sleep apnoea in children include obesity, neuromuscular disorders, craniofacial abnormalities and adenotonsillar hypertrophy.

43) c.
This autosomal recessive disorder is the most common genetic disease in the west.

44) a.
Risk factors for developing leukaemia include high-dose radiation, exposure to the carcinogen benzene and the presence of genetic disorders, in particular Down's syndrome. Chemotherapy is the mainstay of treatment.

45) a.

46) a.
The Guthrie test is specific for the detection of phenylketonuria. This is a autosomal recessive genetic disorder leading to a build-up of the amino acid phenylalanine due to a deficiency of the hepatic enzyme phenylalanine hydroxylase. In the UK, the heel-prick test is a screen for the genetic disorders listed in the options above. The Guthrie test is part of the heel-prick test.

47) e.

48) c.
This condition is the most common hip problem in adolescence.

49) b.
Scarlet fever is caused by *Streptococcus pyogenes*, a group A streptococcus.

50) d.

5. Paediatrics: EMQ Answers

1) A.
Koplik's spots are seen before the measles rash.

2) F.
This is a patient with glandular fever and upper airway obstruction.

3) E.
This is also known as fifth disease and is caused by parvovirus B19. Infection with this virus can cause aplastic crisis in patients with sickle cell disease.

4) C.

5) I.
Treatment includes high-dose aspirin initially and then a lower dose for 6–8 weeks to prevent thrombotic events. Intravenous IgG is also administered in the initial stages and has been shown to reduce the rates of coronary artery aneurysm.

6) B.
Cystic fibrosis is diagnosed by an abnormally high sweat chloride level.

7) A.
Coeliac disease is suggested by a mixed anaemia (iron and folic acid deficiencies). However the definitive diagnosis is made by biopsy of the jejunum.

8) F.
This is a case of hyperthyroidism.

9) J.
This is a case of juvenile-onset diabetes mellitus.

10) I.
The four classic signs of congestive heart failure include tachycardia, tachypnoea, cardiomegaly and hepatomegaly.

11) C.
A CT scan of the head is unnecessary in the absence of signs of increased intracranial pressure. A skull radiograph to look for skull fracture is more than adequate.

12) D.

Non-accidental injury should be considered here. A chest radiograph to exclude rib fractures is required.

13) H.

This child is experiencing signs of increased intracranial pressure with hypertension and bradycardia. For a 2 year old, the resting heart rate should be >95 beats/min. The blood pressure is too high for a 2 year old.

14) D.

In a 2 year old, an AP chest view will more than adequately image the neck and chest to reveal a radio-opaque coin lodged in the cricopharyngeal region.

15) D.

This 4 year old should be investigated for left basal pneumonia. She clearly has diaphragmatic irritation. The edge of the kidney is being irritated, leading to leakage of red blood cells. This is an actual patient case!

16) C.

The patient has coeliac disease.

17) A.

The patient has developed pseudomembranous colitis, which is treated with vancomycin or metronidazole.

18) E.

The baby has intussusception. This can be both diagnosed and treated by barium enema. However, the mortality rate is still 1% due to delays in diagnosis and treatment.

19) F.

This baby may have Hirschsprung's disease, which is confirmed by rectal biopsy.

20) G.

This patient most probably has Wilson's disease and should avoid copper-containing foods.

21) A.

Surfactant is produced by type II pneumocytes, specialized cells within the lung. Surfactant helps to prevent the collapse of alveoli.

22) D.

23) G.

Respiratory syncytial virus (RSV) is the cause of bronchiolitis in over half of all presentations.

24) B.

This is an inherited disorder. α_1-Antitrypsin is an enzyme produced by the liver and stops the degeneration of lung tissue by the enzyme neutrophil elastase. A deficiency of α_1-antitrypsin results in destruction of lung tissue and consequently emphysema develops. In some patients a nominal amount of the enzyme is produced but this is usually defective and accumulates in the liver causing liver damage.

25) C.